A Layperson's Guide to

LIVING
WITH
Mental Disease

By Kathie Maier Rodkey

A LAYPERSON'S GUIDE TO LIVING WITH MENTAL DISEASE

© 2021 Kathie Maier Rodkey

ISBN PRINT 978-1-09837-671-0 | ISBN eBOOK 978-1-09837-672-7

CONTENTS

INTRODUCTION

I believe that Mental Disease is the result of biochemical and neurological disorders in the brain caused by hereditary factors or injury to the brain. I believe that until a person suffering from Mental Disease is stabilized on a medication which helps the brain, therapy will not help. I believe that people who have succeeded in living with mental illness, either their own or that of a family member, are valuable resources in helping others deal with the disease. I believe masking Mental Disease symptoms with pot, cocaine and/or alcohol, prevents medications prescribed for depression, Bipolar and other chemical brain disorders from working properly. I have formulated these beliefs over more than a half century of experience and research.

I do not have degrees which would make me an expert in treating people who are mentally ill, but what I do have is experience. For the first 18 years of my life, I lived with my mother, who was diagnosed with Bipolar and Schizophrenia. In the throes of a major nervous breakdown at age 23, she killed two of her children and was intent on murdering three others. At the age of six, I witnessed her do this. I also suffered from depression my entire life. Many other people I am related to have been impacted by this horrible disease. In addition, I have spent over 50 years talking to people plagued with mental problems. It is still not an acceptable practice to use people who know what it is like to walk in the shoes of a person with a brain dysfunction, to help other people going through the same thing. Society still views Mental Disease as a STIGMA, and the result is that many people who are mentally ill are embarrassed to admit they suffer from it or to talk about it.

Mental illness and its associated tendency toward addictions are diseases of the brain, every bit as devastating as cancer and all of the other thousands of maladies which plague the human race. The difference between being mentally ill and having cancer is that people still believe symptoms like sadness, chronic anxiety, sleep and eating issues, suicidal thoughts, fatigue, mania, and on and on, do not constitute a legitimate illness. They tend to think that the afflicted person has brought these issues on themselves and that if they change their behavior or lifestyles they would get better. This attitude has not changed much in the more than 67 years since my mother was diagnosed with Bipolar in 1953.

This guide is an inside look in layman's terms of what it is like to live with someone who is profoundly mentally ill, and what it is like to actually be mentally ill. I am able to discuss what it is like to have brain malfunction from childhood through puberty to adulthood and into old age, having gone through my entire life with the concrete blanket of mental illness over my shoulders. I also hope to help make it easier for people to identify and deal with the complicated process of diagnosing and treating behavioral changes versus Mental Disease.

I started a group on Facebook a few weeks ago called Living with Mental Disease. In that short amount of time, I have added much valuable information to the Guide. I learned that the STIGMA of Mental Disease is as pervasive as it was back in the 1950's. I also realized that people are having a difficult time understanding how mental illness could be a disease of the brain.

I am passionate about the subject of mental illness and believe that it is the most devastating disease of the human body. I wish I could put on one small card all of the information a person needs to help them with Mental Disease, but that is just not possible. In the midst of the heartbreak, confusion, fear, chaos and stress of dealing with a concerning change in personality, people need clearly stated guidelines to follow. I wrote the Guide and developed the Plan of Action, hoping they will be a light in an otherwise dark tunnel to help people maneuver through concerning behavioral changes, having mental illness themselves, or living with and knowing someone with mental illness.

PLAN OF ACTION

The **Plan of Action** is a summary of steps to take to help confirm whether a change in behavior is possibly a mental illness. It can be used for any ages from infant to adolescent to adult. The **Plan of Action** will also be discussed during the individual sections on age.

1. **Do not ignore unusual behavior, hoping it will go away.** Be thorough and aggressive in investigating the situation which might be causing a behavioral issue.

2. **Conduct a thorough body check looking for bruises or anything unusual.** This action is particularly important for an infant, toddler, or other non-verbal adolescent or adult, but just as critical for all children.

3. **Talk to a verbal child, adolescent or adult as soon as possible.** Remain calm and patient and try to obtain any information which might explain the change in behavior.

4. **Assess the home environment.** Address all the issues which might be contributing to behavioral problems. If drugs or alcohol are a factor, this is a critical issue.

5. **Communicate with everyone who cares for your child, adolescent or adult.** Share concerns immediately with these people directly, with supervisors or administrators of a facility, or with law enforcement if warranted.

6. **Schedule a physical exam.** After addressing 1-5 of the Plan of Action without yielding evidence to explain a personality change, a physical exam is necessary to rule out health issues. An example of an illness which can cause anxiety or mood disorders is thyroid disease.

7. **Investigate the family history with regard to mental and physical problems.** Most mental illness has a hereditary component.

8. **Consider a mental health evaluation.** After everything above from 1 to 6 is ruled out and there are still persistent personality changes, then it is possible the behavior might be connected to a mental disorder. If there is a family history of mental illness this must be considered seriously.

9. **Schedule appointment with Psychiatrist.** A Psychiatrist has a medical license to diagnose mental illness and to prescribe medications. A Psychologist uses therapy to help a person with a mental illness function after they are diagnosed.

10. **Medications.** Begin taking drugs prescribed by a Psychiatrist and developed to target areas of the brain which are impaired after conducting extensive brain scans, blood flow activity, and cognitive testing to determine a diagnosis.

11. **Hospitalization.** Often, a person is involuntarily admitted to a hospital after a psychotic break, suicide attempt, harm to others, upon recommendation by a psychiatrist,

or involvement by law enforcement. Sometimes, people voluntarily admit themselves.

12. **Rehabilitation.** Usually occurs when the patient requires long term treatment for mental disorders which are not responding to drug treatment. This situation also includes treatment for substance abuse, which too often is used by people with brain disorders to temporarily make themselves feel better. This also includes therapy, but I believe therapy is not beneficial until the patient is responding to a medication that is working to stabilize the brain.

WHAT IS MENTAL DISEASE?

A disease is defined as a condition of the living animal or plant body or one of its parts that impairs normal functioning and is manifested by distinguishing signs and symptoms.

Mental Disease is a significant change in emotions, thinking and behavior, and not for the better. It results in dysfunction in socializing, working, taking care of a family, and other activities. The brain is an unbelievably complicated organ with millions of circuits controlling all kinds of human functions essential to the quality of life. When any of these circuits misfire or are damaged, bad things happen. When these bad things cannot be explained by physical injuries or illnesses and are chronic (happening every day), Mental Disease is suspected. In other words, circuits in the brain are damaged and this results in the inability of a person to enjoy a functional life. It involves malfunctioning levels of serotonin, dopamine, norepinephrine, and other chemicals in the brain. As a result of the Living with Mental Disease group, I realized I had to explain these chemicals in detail as soon as possible in the Guide.

There are three main chemical neurotransmitters in the brain. Neurotransmitters carry important messages to all of the millions of circuits in the brain by way of the nerves. When the chemical neurotransmitters in the brain are working properly, they allow a person to experience the wonderful joy of being alive. Unfortunately, things go wrong with the human body and diseases occur. Cancer is caused by abnormal cell activity and when it occurs, it gets plenty of attention along with most other diseases. Sadly, mental illness has not been recognized as the legitimate disease of the brain it is.

9

People mistakenly believe that a person exhibiting behavior they don't understand is somehow responsible for it. I can tell you from experience there is not a single person in the world who would deliberately cause themselves to feel mentally ill in any way. Defective neurotransmitters in the brain do not only cause mental problems, they can also be responsible for many serious health issues.

SEROTONIN is the neurotransmitter responsible for sending signals from one part of the nervous system to another. If it is too low, it can result in depression, anxiety, insomnia, and negative thoughts from mild to psychotic (totally out of touch with reality). If it is too high it can result in muscle rigidity and seizures.

NOREPHINEPHRINE is the neurotransmitter responsible for releasing substances to help with the skeletal muscles and heart contractions. This is critical in regulating the flight or fight syndrome and helping people cope with acute threats. If it is too low, it results in depression, anxiety, PTSD (Post Traumatic Stress Syndrome), and substance abuse. If too high, it can result in panic attacks, hyperactivity, euphoria, and high blood pressure.

DOPAMINE is the neurotransmitter which regulates the pleasure center of the brain. If it is not functioning properly, a person can lose the ability to focus, plan, strive and generally find any interest or pleasure in all aspects of life.

Only a PSYCHIATRIST is licensed and trained to diagnose mental disease and prescribe medications to treat what he finds. An Advanced Practice Psychiatric Nurse can also prescribe medications, with or without the approval of a Psychiatrist depending on the state regulations. If a person is low or high in one or more of the basic neurotransmitters, it becomes a delicate dance to prescribe the right medications in the right amounts to help the person. Even if only one chemical is off, it is still a challenge.

Clinical diagnoses of Mental Disease includes Mood Disorders (Depression and Bi-polar), Anxiety Disorders, Personality Disorders (Borderline Personality Disorders considered to be the most painful including Narcissism, Sociopath, and Schizophrenia), Eating Disorders (Bulimia, Anorexia), Trauma Disorders (PTSD), and Substance Abuse (alcohol, drugs). Autism has also been added to a clinical diagnosis of Mental Disease. These will be discussed in detail later on in the guide.

The major warning signs of Mental Disease are chronic long lasting depression (sadness), lack of motivation or enthusiasm (refusing to do anything), insomnia (sleeping too much or too little), isolation (social withdrawal), paranoia (everyone is against me), hearing voices (schizophrenia), moods from high to low (bi-polar), suicidal thoughts, anorexia (starving) and bulimia (binging), anger (toward themselves or others), guilt (I am the reason for all bad things), anxiety (afraid of everything, won't leave house, extreme nervousness, confusion, irritability, walking around in circles, irrational thinking, poor judgement, risky behavior (both sexual and other), constant drinking and use of drugs. Anxiety can exist without depression, however, depression usually includes anxiety.

Some of the behaviors which are mentioned above do occur in pre-pubescence and puberty and can be difficult to separate from Mental Disease. This is why people living with a troubled pubescent or teen sometimes need help to do what is best. The ages from teenager to the mid-twenties is a critical time in assessing mental illness and will be discussed in greater detail in those sections.

Chronic sadness (depression) is the leading symptom of Mental Disease. Finding no joy in life on a continuing basis is a serious problem. There are parts of the brain which when working properly send signals which allow for functional behavior. When these neurotransmitters are out of whack, the brain becomes a person's worst enemy. **Imagine walking in the most beautiful place on Earth (and there are a lot of them) and feeling only that the experience is pointless and makes no sense. It actually feels painful to be alive. Think about the worst day ever and the emotions of hopelessness, fear, sadness, anger, confusion, and nervousness which might have accompanied that time. Now multiply those feelings tenfold and realize they would be there every single day of life. The only time there might be some relief is during sleep, and even getting rest is elusive. Opening the eyes upon waking and being hit with the demons, as I refer to them, knowing they are still there and will have to be dealt with for another lousy day is the worst feeling in the world. This is Mental Disease.**

The type of Mental Disease, the age of the person, hereditary factors, the treatment being received if any, and day-to-day stresses, all combine to determine the length of time it might take to stabilize a person. People spend years searching for the right medications to help them become functional. Unfortunately, some turn to drugs and alcohol, especially those who have Addiction Disorders, which is an illness under the umbrella of Mental Disease. People believe it is easier to get high, even though it is only temporary and enhances the symptoms of the mental illness. Others disappear into a black hole where suicide becomes a constant thought and sometimes an eventual reality.

I will probably reiterate this again and again that I believe
Mental Disease is the most critical health issue of our time and that
it is overwhelming the mental health system.

THE STIGMA

Back in the 1930's, 1940's (the decade when I was born) and 1950's, cancer was considered a sickness to be ashamed of. Ignorant people actually believed that the disease was a result of weakness, lack of moral values, and was contagious. It wasn't even included as a cause of death in obituaries. Over the years, we completely accepted cancer as a "real" disease, but mental illness has remained in the dark ages with regard to being a stigma. When I started my group on Facebook in February of 2021, I realized just how bad the stigma of mental illness still is.

People were actually afraid to even ask questions on my public post for fear others would think they were mentally ill themselves. Some said they wouldn't join the group for the same reason. I was accused of being callous and even of exploiting people, although no names have been used in either the Guide or the group. There is pervasive fear and misunderstanding about Mental Disease.

The most outrageous offense to Mental Disease is the refusal on the part of people to acknowledge that it is an actual disease, every bit as legitimate as cancer and all the other diseases of the body. To add insult to injury, to this day it is still considered shameful when someone has mental issues. It even impacts a person's ability to get a job, as they are often seen as unfit. Many professional people, including Psychiatrists and Psychologists, will not reveal that they have mental issues themselves for fear of losing patients. It is ironic, because I truly believe that a doctor who has dealt with personal mental issues makes a much more understanding and empathetic person to treat someone else with mental issues.

Nothing has changed if young people struggling with depression today still won't admit they are sick, and their family doesn't acknowledge it either. If a child has cancer, it is shared with the word for help and support, but if the prognosis has the word mental in it, it is immediately treated like the plague. There is not much sympathy and understanding for the fact that Mental Disease is a misfiring of circuits in the brain which need fixing, just like the cancer cells which invade the bodies of humans.

One of my grandchildren did an extensive report about the stress on athletes to be physically strong, with basically no attention paid to their mental well-being. Nobody wants to talk about mental health, and again the shame factor prevents athletes and other people from seeking help. Our entire culture pushes being strong as a measure of success. It is no surprise that a person suffering from depression or other mental disorders would keep it to themselves, when society does not accept or view mental illness as the legitimate disease it is.

In 1953, I overheard one of my relatives say, "We can't keep her with us. She has to go someplace else. I will be fired from my job if they find out that was my sister who killed her kids." I was the "her" he was referring to not keeping and I was out of his house by early the next morning. Not one person in my family talked about my mother or what she did, as if it never happened. To this day, people still hide or feel they can't talk about their mental problems. This pervasive attitude has and will continue to be the greatest obstacle to making any significant headway with Mental Disease.

Because of the stigma of Mental Disease, the patriarch of a certain famous family ordered a lobotomy for his child when he saw signs of mental illness. The procedure went wrong and left the child unable to walk or talk. The child most likely had depression or bipolar and did not require that type of extreme therapy, but in this case the shame of mental illness drove the family to a tragic treatment decision. A lobotomy involved severing connections in the prefrontal cortex of the brain. The last lobotomy was done in 1967 and resulted in the patient's death. The procedure was banned and is no longer performed.

HEREDITY

There are many illnesses in the human race that are hereditary. For example, Cystic Fibrosis can occur when both the mother and father are carriers. Back in the day, no one paid much attention to DNA, and actually pushed most of the uncomfortable information about family illnesses under the proverbial rug. In today's day and age, there are many tests to help couples determine whether future children might be at risk for certain devastating diseases. Determining the risk for a child having a mental illness does not have a concrete test like other diseases, although some high technology brain scans can shed light on areas of the brain which are not working properly. Radioactive tracers in Perfusion SPECT brain scans can show the extent of neurological impairment in the brain connected with Mental Disease, Traumatic Brain Injury (TBI), and frontal and temporal lobe issues. A regular CAT scan and MRI only show basic anatomical problems, and sometimes miss even those.

I believe strongly that even people who incur mental illness after serious brain injuries or later in life, have a hereditary component in their brain that makes mental illness more likely. If that wasn't the case, everyone who had a brain injury or was entering old age, would also have mental illness. This is certainly not the case. If the chemical activity in the brain is subject to changes due to brain injury or getting older, this is most likely hereditary.

Helping family members who are in trouble from mental issues, requires honesty about the family history and a willingness to be aggressive in investigating and talking about mental illness. This is not high on anyone's list, considering the stigma of Mental

Disease. It is somewhat likely that a descendent might inherit Mental Disease if one grandparent or parent are mentally ill. It is highly likely, especially if both parents and grandparents are mentally ill. If mental illness is rampant among many family members on both sides of the family, there is reason to be concerned about the mental health of future descendants. When assessing reasons why a child or adult might be suffering from depression, etc., **the family history is paramount.** From many years of experience, I can say this information is still not easily attainable.

A Psychiatrist who was evaluating a family member's child and reviewing the incidence of mental illness on two sides of the family said, "I have never seen in my entire career a family so profoundly stricken with Mental Disease". He was able to understand more readily why the child was suffering from certain symptoms.

Some mental disorders have a higher degree of hereditary as per scientific research. For instance, Schizoaffective Disorder, definitely does present more in people with an immediate family member who has the disorder. Schizoaffective Disorder manifests with psychotic symptoms such as hallucinations, delusions and mood disorders along with symptoms of depression and mania. There will be more about Mental Disease disorders later in the Guide.

My mother was the youngest of ten children in an Irish Catholic family plagued with mental illness and serious addictions to alcohol and drugs. Long after my mother died, I talked to her only surviving sibling about her. My aunt was a few years older than my mother and was able to describe her as a young child. She said my mother was fragile from the beginning. She was moody, sullen and withdrawn on most days and on other days inappropriately giddy, hyper and involved in risky behavior, which often got her in trouble. She said things got much worse when she started menstruating.

My aunt also confirmed that three of her brothers were mentally ill with addictions. Her oldest brother's six children were put in foster care with disastrous results because he and his wife abandoned them while on an alcoholic bender. Her other two brothers ended up on skid row and died as the result of mental illness, combined with alcohol and drug addiction. One brother was in a drunken stupor, went to the bathroom, pulled the overhead chain too hard and the water closed fell on his head and killed him.

By the time I talked to my aunt about my mother it was 50 plus years later and she knew my mother was bipolar with schizophrenia, but she also revealed that her sisters all had depression, eating disorders and alcohol addictions. Only one aunt and uncle escaped full-blown mental and addiction issues in a family of ten children. The mental illness has not been as pervasive as it was with the aunts and uncles, but all of the ten branches on the family tree have people on them who have inherited Mental Disease and addictive disorders.

My mother's father and mother were both much older when they had my mother, their youngest child. We now know from research that the older parents are when a child is conceived, the more prone that child might be to mental illness. In this case, I don't believe the age of her parents had anything to do with her mental illness, as that would not explain the serious mental issues with the children they had when they were much younger. There was 20 years difference between the first child and the youngest. I believe this is a legitimate example of the impact of heredity on mental well-being. My mother's father was an alcoholic also, but no one talked about mental illness so I was not able to get concrete data on the mental health of the people above my grandfather on the family tree. Unfortunately, many cousins on each branch of the tree inherited Mental Disease and addiction disorders.

I don't know if I was an unhappy child before the age of six. I remember nothing of my life prior to the day I watched my mother kill my two brothers in the midst of a nervous breakdown. The home I lived in was dysfunctional until I moved out at 18. I suffered with depression until I was finally diagnosed during a clinical trial at the age of 60. I should have known I needed help all of those years, but being mentally ill completely throws your judgement off with regard to what you need to do to feel better.

I was blindsided by an early traumatic event, with absolutely no counseling. Actually, there were no child psychiatrists or psychologists at that time. The thought was children should be seen but not heard, and that we didn't have any feelings worth discussing. The psychiatric community had no idea the **GUILT** children feel with regard to many events occurring in their lives would stay with them forever. The guilt I felt about not saving my two brothers tore me up until I confided in a psychiatrist about the situation. She set me straight by proving to me that I would have died on that day if I had tried to help my brothers. I was in my 20's by the time I discussed my guilt and got the information I needed to convince me that I could not have saved my siblings without getting myself killed.

My home environment continued to be stressful and dysfunctional throughout my entire childhood. I did not know my mother was found not guilty by reason of insanity in the deaths of my brothers and the attempted murder of my sister until I was much older. I was completely unaware of the extent of the mental illness on the maternal side of my family until I was in my late 20's. I think it might have helped me if I had known that it wasn't just my mother and myself who were ill, and that I had a very strong hereditary predisposition toward Mental Disease.

Unfortunately, in addition to my mother's family history, my father was not mentally clear either. Who would have five more children with a person who murdered two of his children and was attempting to murder all five of them? Especially after telling a family member that "she killed my favorite child". Who in their right mind would leave a seven year old and other youngsters alone with a person going through a nervous breakdown, when that person had already killed two of his children? And this behavior continued until I left the house at 18. I cannot count the amount of times we kids were left alone with a mother suffering a mental breakdown.

FAMILY

The impact on a family when one of its members is mentally ill is life changing. Some ignore behavioral changes until a catastrophic event demands action. Some obsess totally on the ill person and neglect the rest of the family. Some rely on a single family member to make everything right, putting great pressure on that person. Some work hard to achieve a good balance between taking care of the mentally ill person and preserving the sanity of the rest of the family members. This is the best course of action, but extremely difficult. The havoc a mentally ill person is capable of causing in a household can range from exhaustion, to abuse, to fear, to anger, to sadness, to danger, and worse.

The hardest thing I went through as a child with a mentally ill mother was the pressure that was put on me at such a young age to help her do her job as a mother. The worst thing was the expectation that I would stay with her when she was in the throes of a nervous breakdown, which was often. This was my father's poor judgement, as he had to work to support the expanding family and he never questioned whether I could do it or not. He was just glad to get out the door and go to work. When he came home, everything was usually in order except for those scary times when my mother was completely out of control after days or weeks of slowly and painfully going off the deep end. Those were the times he would take her to the hospital and I would lock the door behind them, with a sigh of relief.

As long my mother was taking her pills faithfully, she did take care of us as best she could with the help of two or three packs of cigarettes a day. The problem was that with her mental illness, the increasing family became more of a burden for her fragile state and she needed more help and suffered more breakdowns. She also was inconsistent taking her medications, another unfortunate side effect of mental illness.

When I came home from school, my mother was usually exhausted. Taking any mental health medication will cause fatigue, but it is worth it when they fix the broken brain. I was expected to help with the younger children and whatever chores needed to be done. I had to make dinner many nights. It was a struggle to get to my homework, and that would be the way it was until I graduated from high school. I never enjoyed learning as I was always rushing through my homework and had a hard time concentrating on what I was hearing in the classroom. I studied hard for tests and always got great grades, but I was not really retaining what I learned. I use geography as an example. Today, I know the map of the world like the back of my hand and thoroughly enjoyed the process of learning where every Continent was. In school, I struggled to retain just what was necessary to pass a test, always thinking about what I would be facing at home. I was trying to cope with my own dysfunctional mental health journey, while taking care of my mother's dysfunction.

My mother's frequent breakdowns resulted in days lost at school. If the episode did not result in her being hospitalized, I could go to school only if my father was home. When she was hospitalized, I missed school until social services came to the rescue. There was no information, so I never knew when I would go back to school. Because of what I went through, I am a firm believer in communication and honesty, especially with a child over six. I needed it badly to allay my fears and anxieties about the future. I never got either. It completely destroyed my trust in people.

I was painfully silent. I had lots to say in my mind, but the words never came out because I felt no one would listen. I shut down verbally immediately after my brothers died. I don't know if I was quiet before then, but that information was never going to be revealed as no one discussed the past. I was sad every single minute of the day. It didn't help that I was going to Catholic school, where the atmosphere was dark to say the least. Even at that, it was still better than being at home. I often wonder, and forgive me if I repeat this again, if having adult responsibilities so young strengthened me to cope better with my own depression throughout the years? Or did never getting to be a child make me more depressed than I would have been? Society needs to think about the stresses which are put on young children with regard to all facets of their lives, even if they believe it is for their own good. A child needs to be a child for as long as possible or it sets them up for future mental health issues.

Family members caring for a mentally ill person are most often emotionally fraught and exhausted from their journey. They are in the position of supporting someone who does not want to or can't cooperate with them on any reasonable level. Their only leverage is the fact that they are supplying a roof over the mentally ill person's head. Often, especially with teenagers and those over 18, they leave the home when rules are given which they don't want to follow. Things get so bad in the home that ultimatums are necessary in order to restore peace, and many families lose their loved ones to the streets. If the mentally ill person has not yet succeeded in getting a medication to help with their specific brain issue, the chances are much higher that they will resist any help from family and will end up homeless, in crack houses, or worse. In many cases, they will refuse to leave and continue to destroy the functional environment in their home.

In any case, when a person or persons in a family are suffering from Mental Disease, the rest of the family must not be ignored. They can often times feel very guilty that they are somehow responsible for the behavior of the mentally ill family member. Issues should be discussed with complete honesty as often as possible. Remember, young children will think the worst if they are confused about what is going on and information is not shared with them. A person cannot be given a pass to abuse family members with word or deed, because of their mental state. The other members of the family should be given support, love, praise, honest information, and thanks as often as possible as they cope with the new dynamic. **Finally, a young person should NEVER be left alone with someone who is mentally ill.**

ISOLATION - A CRITICAL SYMPTOM

Before I start discussing mental illness in the different age groups, I have recently been involved with a situation where the first behavioral change with a young child was social isolation. It reminded me of how important this symptom is. Isolation, or withdrawing from all socialization, is in most cases one of the first concerning personality changes people recognize in a child or adult. Teens going through puberty will often spend lots of time alone in their room and have to be coaxed to eat dinner with or participate in other family functions. They tend to sleep more, but that is because they are up late at night on the phone or on the computer. Also, growth spurts and changing hormones are known to make people more tired. The majority of people experiencing isolation without mental illness, will go to school and participate in extracurricular activities, even though they might have to be encouraged to do so. They will also keep up with their hygiene and might actually even get more obsessive about their grooming.

When a once active and social family member suddenly wants to spend all day in bed, refuses to do anything, stops caring about hygiene, and suffers insomnia at night, they could be sinking into depression. They are usually very uncooperative about resuming normal activity. This symptom cannot be ignored and the **Plan of Action** needs to be started immediately, ruling out a possible physical or external issue causing the problem.

Isolation from family, is an early warning sign of a significant issue in a person, especially if they have always been social. It cannot be ignored, and they must be monitored carefully and encouraged to get help. There are people who are hermits and just don't like socializing and they are otherwise functional in life, but they have a long history of that behavior without negative incidents, and so their families can rest easy that they are not a threat in any way. Sudden withdrawal from socializing as a personality change cannot be ignored.

BEHAVIORAL CHANGES/ MENTAL DISEASE FROM INFANCY TO ADVANCED AGE

As promised, this is the section which will hopefully give important information as to what to expect from the different age groups with regard to determining normal changes in behavior versus changes which could indicate Mental Disease.

NON-VERBAL: INFANCY TO EARLY TODDLER

With the exceptions of mental retardation, which is usually diagnosed before or at birth, and autism, it is rare that a mental illness is found in an infant or toddler. If a child seems sad and withdrawn, has developmental delays, problem making eye contact, eating issues, and inability to mimic facial expressions, the child should be seen by a pediatrician as soon as possible as these are initial symptoms of autism. With autism, the sooner the infant is diagnosed and receives therapy, the better chance they have of overcoming some of their issues.

I cannot talk from personal experience about mental illness in infancy as my depression began at six years old. What I can offer, from talking to people dealing with changes in the behavior of an infant, is the following.

The most frequent concern of young parents with regard to their babies and toddlers is when they experience a personality change from a happy-go-lucky child to a sad, withdrawn one. This is where the Plan of Action comes into play again.

Honestly assessing the home environment is important. Is there ongoing stress? Are there frequent arguments which can be overheard by the child? Is bonding time from one or both parents limited? Does the child spend long hours away from home with a caretaker? Does the child get limited stimulation? I have seen toddlers who cannot speak spend hours on a cell phone or IPad, amusing themselves. To me, every hour a non-verbal child is not interacting with other human beings, cannot be good. The jury is still out on the long-term issues of constant technology, but already there are studies which indicate that sadness and depression are being diagnosed in people who spend more time in front of computers and video games. Also, there are more incidents of mental illness in younger children than ever before.

For non-verbal children, the only way of expressing pain or unhappiness is by crying or becoming sad and withdrawn. These are dark times and we cannot trust anyone when it comes to our children. It is not possible when a child is an infant or non-verbal toddler to teach or talk to them about inappropriate touching, so a parent must be vigilant and aggressive in paying attention to a personality change or bodily injuries. As a matter of fact, even if a child seems normal it is a good idea to check them often when they return from caretakers. A good caretaker will inform a parent if a child has fallen or had an issue which resulted in a bruise or cut.

If a child has unusual bruises or marks on any part of the body which cannot be explained, take the child to a pediatrician as soon as possible. The specialist will look for health issues which might explain sudden bruises, but if the doctor feels there is evidence of abuse, the law requires the authorities to be called.

It is essential to rule out whether a child is being physically or verbally abused or bullied by an adult, another child, or even a family pet or other animal outside the home. A visit to the home or facility where the child is cared for is in order if anything is suspected. Stay calm, patient and be thorough when talking to the child's caretakers and scoping out the environment. Sometimes, a non-verbal child will tell by their actions if they are uncomfortable with someone or something. They might stiffen up or cling tightly, look away from the caretaker, or start crying as if they want to get away. If parents are aggressive with their investigations, they should be able to determine if a child is being abused verses having behavioral changes due to a possible mental illness.

Everything in the first part of the **Plan of Action** has been ruled out, but the infant or toddler continues to be sad and withdrawn or agitated. If the child has not had a checkup as part of the process above, then it is time to explore whether a physical issue might be causing the change. For example, the child could have an allergy causing pain or itching or the thyroid could be malfunctioning, which causes anxiety and mood changes. To repeat, if the child is having other developmental delays, an autism check is warranted. Children who are born to drug addicts and alcoholics are also more susceptible to personality changes. Generally, as they withdraw from drugs, the mood improves, but not always if the damage is severe. Studies have shown that these children might also be more susceptible to Mental Disease if the brain circuits have been damaged.

If all of the above has been explored and the baby is still not as happy as you would like, it is possible the child's personality has changed to resemble that of an in-law! Hopefully, the personality will change again. Sorry, I can't help it! A sense of humor is critical especially in these times.

Continue to keep a close eye on the child, but don't obsess over it once everything has been ruled out. Many babies and toddlers go through personality changes from time to time. Continue to provide a happy, stress-free environment and never argue in front of a child of any age. If you know that there are mental issues among family members, vigilance is more important as the child ages, especially if the melancholy doesn't subside or worsens. Eventually, the child will become verbal and will hopefully be able to communicate what they are feeling.

VERBAL TODDLER TO FIVE YEARS

I wish I could say that full blown Mental Disease is rarely seen in this group of children, but unfortunately that is not true. There have been cases of four and five year olds consistently doing harm to themselves and others in the throes of severe anger issues. Years later, and while they are still children, extensive brain scans have shown that the Hippocampus and Amygdala and other part of their brains which control emotions were severely damaged. If the Amygdala is sending destructive messages to the Hippocampus, a child as young as five years old could easily stab several members of his family without thinking twice about it. Unfortunately, it does happen and the violence can continue until they are diagnosed. Some families endure this horror for a decade or longer before they get help. Some never get relief.

A SPECT brain scan was performed on the five year old who stabbed his relatives, but it didn't happen until he was 15 and had caused his family a decade of the most unbelievable stress imaginable. The test did confirm that his brain was damaged in many areas, especially those neurotransmitters controlling anger and impulsiveness. With the help of a Psychiatrist and the right medications targeted to the dysfunctional areas of his brain, he might finally get the help he needs. **Many people cannot believe that the brain of a five-year old can be that damaged, but with the right mix of heredity,**

birth trauma, a possible brain injury, and environmental factors it can happen.

There are many tests available to help determine the functioning of the brain. MRI and PET scans are the most popular and are usually covered by insurance. They are useful but sometimes do not show everything that is needed to diagnose the patient. The SPECT (single-photon emission computerized tomography) brain scan has been very successful in showing where abnormal functioning is taking place in the brain. It is a nuclear imaging test using radioactive materials and a camera to create 3-D pictures. This test which costs about $1300 is not covered by insurance because they have determined that attention deficit is a behavioral problem. Behavioral problems are not deemed eligible for coverage by insurance. Many mental health professionals do not believe the SPECT makes any difference in a diagnosis, but a desperate parent looking for answers to a loved one's mental health crisis may disagree with that assessment. I disagree wholeheartedly with the insurance companies also and believe SPECT brain scans will be the wave of the future to diagnose mental illness.

I will never forget visiting a teenager in a rehabilitation center. I was ready to get on the elevator, when the door opened and out walked at least ten children, all of whom were no more than five or six years old. After I inquired if they were patients, one of the people working in the facility told me the children were being moved from one therapy session to another. I felt the tears leave my eyes and I had the chills for a long time.

It is hoped that even if there is no change of personality with a verbal child, that the important subject of inappropriate touching has already taken place. This is probably the most sensitive and critical talk which people need to have with a young child.

There are books and other educational materials to help family communicate the issue in the best way. It also includes making sure the child knows that they have done nothing wrong when an adult touches them inappropriately, as feeling guilty about everything bad which takes place is rampant among children. They have to be reassured they can come to a parent and tell them what is happening immediately no matter what it is. People need to tell children that people who are doing bad things to them will often tell them they can't say anything about it or will even threaten them or their family. Too many people don't want to discuss "upsetting" issues with their children. They want their children to believe the world is a rosy place to live, and keep them in a bubble. Remember, children will feed off of anxiety or other emotions they feel from an adult. In some cases, they are more perceptive than adults. Many children won't tell the truth no matter how often they are questioned, mainly because of overwhelming guilt or fear, so that has to be taken into account. Again, it is a sad state of affairs that we have to deal with issues like this at such an early age, but it is better than the lifelong ramifications of having a child who has been abused repeatedly and is too naïve, guilty or afraid to sound the alarm.

For children in this age group who are experiencing behavioral changes, the Plan of Action is a valuable tool. The difference from non-verbal children is that the child in this age group is communicating, so hopefully it makes it a lot easier to find out what might be happening. In some cases, the situation could become even more complicated depending on the answers to questions and how cooperative the child is.

Talking to the child, calmly and patiently, is the first order of business. Focus on whether they have any problems with the home environment, assuring the child that no matter what they say they are safe. A parent should help the child by bringing up things they themselves feel might be bothering the child, like frequent arguments. If it is not too overwhelming in one discussion, ask them questions about their caretakers, schools, friends, other family members, neighbors, and even the family pet to determine if there is abuse or bullying. If the child becomes agitated by any specific question, it might indicate this is where the problem lies.

You may wonder why I talk about family pets or other animals, but I have experienced several cases were a child was severely bitten and even killed by a family pet and it was discovered that the animal had been tormenting the child before the alleged incidents. There are also cases where a child tormented the animal, and it bit back. One child lost her nose to the family pet. A child should never be left alone in a room with an animal. Granted, the majority of family pets do not attack children, but when they do it can be a lifelong trauma for the entire family.

There is no question that an examination of the child's body is necessary when the personality changes. There may be nothing evident, but it still has to be done. During a bath, giving the child a washcloth to clean their own private area and reminding them that only they can touch that part of their body sometimes results in the child admitting someone is touching them inappropriately. Of course, any redness, swelling or rashes seen in private areas or identified by the child must be followed up immediately by a Pediatrician.

Again, even though I have no personal experience with regard to mental illness from toddler to age five, as my depression started at age six, I can tell you that I know of hundreds of people who have experienced issues with their children at that age, most of which did not turn out to be mental health issues. Many were the result of abuse and/or bullying and were resolved quickly, as by this time the child can verbalize what is happening to them. There were some cases which were directly due to the family environment, including divorce, relocation, illnesses and/or deaths. A few were the result of a delayed Autism diagnosis, which is a part of the mental health disorders. One child had a liver tumor, and another child had a thyroid disease. That is why a complete wellness exam is always a necessity when a child's personality changes.

I do know from talking to occupational, speech and physical therapists that they do treat children under five who have been referred by Psychiatrists for autism issues, anxiety, depression and mania, mostly due to childhood trauma, birth issues, heredity, or serious physical injury to the brain. Again, I will never forget the shock I felt seeing all those little ones getting off of the elevator to go to mental therapy sessions.

I have always taken solace in my belief that being under the age of reason might prevent most children from remembering terrible traumatic events. There are exceptions to every rule, but I like to think the brain which has not reached the age of reason, keeps these terrors from being remembered. For the sake of the many horribly abused, innocent and suffering children, I hope this is true. On the other hand, if a child continues to experience trauma past the age of reason, it is known to cause monumental mental and physical health repercussions during their life.

I have two personal examples of why I believe children under six are less likely to remember traumatic events or feel guilt.

First, my brother was only five when my mother killed my brothers. I don't honestly know if he saw my mother actually throw his brothers out the window, even though he was standing right next to me. I do know for a fact that he does not remember anything about that day, so if he did see it his mind buried it. For me, at six years old, it is the first day of my life. I remember nothing of what came before. My brother went to live with my grandparents during the time my family was separated. My father was living with his parents also, so my brother got to see his dad every day. He remembers nothing of that time either. He seemed very happy when the family reunited. As a matter of fact, I can remember being very upset and jealous that my mother, father, brother and little sister seemed very happy, while I was sad and scared.

Second, a neighbor caught my 15-month old sister as she was thrown from the window, saving her life. My sister was placed in a Catholic foundling home. She remembered nothing of that time. She told me the first memory of her life was when she was seven years old and was missing for hours. She and her friend went up on the roof of the building where we lived, and the exit door locked so they couldn't get out. It was the first traumatic event in her life, and at 7 years old she remembered it well. This represents another example of why most children under five may not remember much of their lives prior to the age of reason. There are exceptions to every rule, and I have heard them all whether they are imagined or real memories. I do believe that the brain does protect the innocent from remembering horrible things which are done to them before the age of reason. I can feel a little bit better believing this is the case, especially in view of the amount of abuse which happens involving children.

There is a difference with children today that worries mental health professionals, and that is the frequent access to technology. I have seen so many very young children, even infants and toddlers, playing with cell phones and IPads for long periods of time. Aside from the fact that they are not running around getting exercise and stimulation, I wonder what it is doing to their developing brain. It certainly limits communication with the people in their lives and that is already becoming a problem. One of the key symptoms of Autism is the inability of the person to make direct contact others with their eyes. Unfortunately, children who spend much of their time staring at a screen are exhibiting the same inability to look a person in the face when they are communicating. This is some very unsettling information. With mental illness increasing among young children, I am sure there are studies going on with regard to how the preoccupation with technology could be impacting that increase.

Again, with the exception of autism, birth defects and mental retardation, even though cases of mental illness in very young children are not as frequent, nothing should be ruled out until the Plan of Action has been totally explored.

I hope I have not disappointed anyone who is having serious problems with a child five and under, and that the above suggestions will help. I have already started a group on Living with Mental Disease to help people with questions which are not answered in the Guide.

THE AGE OF REASON: SIX YEARS OLD TO 12

The age of reason refers to a time in human development when the brain is advanced enough to remember events that happen. There will be exceptions, but scientists have determined that six years old is the age when children will most likely remember what happens with clarity, and especially if they are traumatic events. This is also the age when children start to internalize guilt when something goes wrong, even if it is not their fault. It is connected to brain development and the ego and really manifests itself more when they are six and older. This is the time when my personal experience with mental illness began.

I was lying in a strange bed, with a cousin on either side of me. *"My stomach hurt so badly. People were whispering, but I could still hear what they were saying, and they didn't want me around. Why did my grandmother slap me in the face when I picked up the newspaper with the pictures of my two brothers on it? What did I do wrong? I must have done something bad to cause all of this. Where is the rest of my family? They all must hate me and that is why I am alone? My head hurts and I feel like throwing up, but I can't move or I will get in trouble, and I don't want to be in any more trouble."*

I will remember until I die the panic I experienced as a six year old watching my mother kill my siblings, knowing she was doing something wrong but not processing the enormity of it. I know exactly what happens when a situation is so frightening that the person becomes paralyzed with inaction. I felt instantly hot and cold and faint. My feet felt like they were stuck in mud. Then my mother looked right at me with those demon eyes as she reached for my little sister, jarring me into action. I grabbed my brother's hand and dragged him out of the room.

The above represents the first memories of my life on Earth.

On that day, I was ripped apart from my family. I didn't know for a very long time, and well after childhood, that my ensuing sadness, unhappiness, guilt, fear, depression, anxiety, paranoia, lack of trust, non-existent self-esteem and physical problems were the result of a devastating trauma, abandonment, non-existent counseling, and a serious family history of mental illness

I went into survival mode, trying to make it from minute to minute. Five minutes drinking a small glass of soda with a cookie to dip in it given to me by a sympathetic aunt was heaven. A bed to sleep in, even though there were five other kids in it, meant one more night of survival. An extra piece of white bread with sugar and butter on it from the wonderful people who hosted me during the summer was a victory. I managed to get through my sixth year, but surviving got much more complicated as I got older.

I hope by telling you about what I went through at each stage of my struggle with mental illness, it will give you more confidence about my experience and suggestions. I walked the walk, living with someone mentally ill and being mentally ill myself, and I believe with all my heart that experience is the best teacher.

Today, anyone who is dealing with someone whose personality has changed and not for the better, has resources available to them. Unfortunately, there can be a lot of emotion and confusion about where to begin, no matter how old a person is. Again, the **Plan of Action** needs to be followed.

What is the difference between a sad, unhappy baby, toddler or child under five versus a child over six years old?

Back in the day, there was no difference because it was believed that children were not capable of feeling anything. They were seen but not heard, and so there was no thought of counseling if behavior changed. Actually, child Psychiatrists or Psychologists did not even exist for children. Nowadays, the increase in mental illness among children is rampant. Because a six year old is definitely forming lasting memories of life, it becomes even more critical to get to the bottom of what might be causing their issues. At six and older, children become more social, attending school, parties, and extracurricular activities. With increased socialization, the possibility of events causing personality changes increases. In most cases, they are temporary forks in the road, but cannot be ignored.

A formerly very happy child, becomes difficult, sullen, withdrawn, quiet, angry and/or sad. They may stop grooming themselves completely, isolate themselves in their rooms, have no interest in family activities, refuse to do homework, antagonize everyone, and don't want to talk. The **Plan of Action** for ruling out what could be causing the change is basically the same for all ages, with the exception that in this stage the child is verbal and might be able to help solve the mystery, or just make it more frustrating with stubborn silence.

Following the **Plan of Action**, the change in personality has not been ignored. The child has been checked for obvious signs of abuse, as much as they will allow, and asked directly about inappropriate touching by anyone. Females asking females questions about their bodies and males asking males about their bodies, as children this age are very reluctant to want even parents looking at their bodies.

Additional discussions have been held with the child, covering issues in the home like frequent arguments, separation, divorce, relocations, long work hours, illness or recent deaths. Patience and calmness has been maintained, allowing the child to confide anything which might be going on not only at home, but in school, on the playground, at a friend's home, during activities or any place else they frequent. Remembering always, that children this age do feel guilty about everything and will often clam up about anything they are going through. If necessary, investigations have been conducted with caretakers, the school, or any other environments to rule out concerns which still exist after discussion with the child.

If none of the above results in a plausible explanation for a troubled, sad child, then the next step is a thorough physical exam. As was explained previously, there are many disorders other than mental illness which can change a child's personality. A physical exam is essential to rule out illnesses, such as thyroid diseases or tumors, which can cause anxiety and mood disorders. If a definite illness is diagnosed by the child's Pediatrician and confirmed by a second opinion, and that explains the personality change, the Pediatrician will continue caring for his patient. If, however, there is no physical cause, **I do not recommend that a Pediatrician treat any child for what they believe is a mental illness such as anxiety, bipolar or depression.** Unless the Pediatrician is a licensed Psychologist also, they should not be recommending a mental health medication to a child. I know of several very bad outcomes when children were given prescriptions for anxiety or other mental health issues by a doctor other than a Psychiatrist. Some side effects are very catastrophic if the drug is not administered correctly and monitored vigilantly.

I firmly believe from past experience that Mental Disease must be treated by mental health experts, such as Psychiatrists and Psychologists. A Psychiatrist is a medical doctor who is licensed to both diagnose and prescribe medications for Mental Disease and talk to the patient about medication management. Psychologists focus on treating emotional and mental suffering in patients already diagnosed with a mental illness, using psychotherapy and behavioral intervention. They do not prescribe drugs. The more specialized they are, the better they will be able to help your child. Medications for mental diseases should only be prescribed by professionals who are experts in specific diagnosis. The side effects can be complicated, and close monitoring is required. Again, I believe if there is money for a brain scan then that becomes the first priority for a diagnosis which will lead to the right medication and therapy.

Keep in mind, children are entering puberty earlier than they have in the past, so a child 12 or under could be experiencing changes in hormone and testosterone levels resulting in personality differences. I believe the ages from puberty to the mid-twenties are the worst for the onset of Mental Disease. I will be discussing this further in the sections dealing with those ages, but I want to make sure parents keep in mind the fact that puberty can happen in some children 12 and under and could be a plausible reason for a change in personality.

Also, at this point I need to address the subject of guilt. I can say with complete confidence that **guilt is something all children feel**, whether they are prone to mental illness or not. After the release of my book, *Free To Be Insane*, I had occasion to talk to young children who had experienced trauma of many different kinds such as assault, physical and verbal abuse, divorce, death, accidents, etc. The one thing that was common for almost all of them was they felt they were responsible for what happened, even if they were in no way culpable. I cannot stress enough the importance of a child being counseled about changing events in their lives, whether they are catastrophic or not, to make sure they do not feel guilty about anything. Chronic guilt can tear a child to pieces.

I felt tremendous guilt from the age of six to my mid-twenties that I had not tried to save my brothers. A Psychiatrist I worked for told me after hearing and investigating my story, that I probably would not have survived trying to save my brothers from my mother. She encouraged me to write down my story for cathartic relief. More than half a century later, I read in newspaper accounts that I was considered a hero for saving my brother. I also found out that in her psychotic state, my mother would have picked me up like a rag doll and thrown me out of the window. It took five firemen to restrain her. If someone had told me all of that immediately after the tragedy, maybe it would have made a difference in my overall mental state and saved me from all of those years of guilt. It certainly couldn't have hurt. The deck was stacked against me though, as children were seen but not heard during that period of time.

Did the early trauma I suffered cause me to become a more sullen, depressed, anxious and complicated person? Did the fact that my mother's entire family plagued with mental illness and addictions, mean that I was destined for follow in their footsteps? Did the fact that I was abandoned by my family for a long time and then returned to a dysfunctional family dynamic for more than a decade after, accelerate the tendency toward mental disease? I believe so.

The above is why it is so important to follow the Plan of Action to give a child or an adult suffering with personality or mental problems the best chance to have quality of life as soon as possible. Maybe if I had honest communication from the adults in my life and had not been abandoned for so long, or been in a safe environment where I felt comfortable, accepted, and loved, I would not have suffered depression so soon and so badly. On the other hand, maybe my hereditary predisposition was so strong I would have become mentally ill very early no matter how great my childhood was. I don't think so, and that is why I believe it is so important for children to have stress-free childhoods filled with fun. I firmly believe the neurotransmitters and chemicals in the brain rear their ugly heads sooner if a child is under constant stress. It is one of the reasons why Mental Disease among young people is increasing.

There are millions of depressed people who are living with other mentally ill people, and that complicates the quality of life for everyone involved. This is the time to talk about my living with a mentally ill mother for 18 years, while coping with my own depression.

My mother was found not guilty by reason of insanity for killing the boys and the attempted murder of my little sister. She was remanded to a psychiatric institution. I was placed with one of my mother's sisters, who had six children of her own. She got me into a social services program for the summer, and I was sent to live with the host family. They were good to me, but no matter what they did from bread and sugar sandwiches to picnics and swimming, I found it impossible to smile or be happy. I remember I did not want to go home when the time came, but I know it was a pleasant experience and I felt very comfortable with them. During that time, I never got any information about my family and I didn't have the nerve to ask. I was practically a mute, speaking only when spoken too.

My mother was released from the psychiatric hospital in less than a year. My father, mother, brother and little sister, showed up at the home of the most recent person I was staying with, a neighbor of one of my relatives. I was panic stricken and afraid for my life. I wanted to ask them so many things, but no words escaped my mouth. I wanted them to talk about my little brothers, but that never happened.

The day they picked me up, we moved into a third floor apartment. I was sick to my stomach and upset that everyone seemed so happy. The bedroom for my sister and I had the window with the fire escape outside of it, so I felt instantly relieved that my mother would not be able to throw us out easily. My brother was in a bedroom by himself with a window that had no protection and a straight drop to the concrete below. I didn't envy him at all.

I was now 7 years old. I began eating dirt, a lot of it, from the sides of buildings and underneath cars. I also ate chalk and the lead from pencils. There are several theories for this eating disorder from an iron deficiency to a chemical imbalance in the brain which causes odd habits. I just know I craved it and it actually tasted good. The only reason I stopped was because I was afraid of getting caught. I was also putting a kitchen butter knife under my pillow every night to protect myself, just in case my mother decided to hurt me. Serious insomnia and sleep issues are a huge problem for people with mental illness. It took me hours to go to sleep as my mind was constantly turning with scenarios for my demise. Opening my eyes every morning was a painful experience. My world was dark and dreary, without joy. I remember feeling completely sad when I heard a plane flying overhead. I felt so lonely and hopeless. I still have flashbacks to those times, especially when I hear an airplane.

The only thing that got me up every day was the fact that I was getting out of the house to go to school. My brother and I were enrolled in a Catholic school, tuition paid for by the Diocese. I hated it. The nuns and priests were mean, but it was still better than being at home. So I eagerly went to school and worked to get good grades, the only thing I had some control over, and which made me feel better about myself. This need to excel continued throughout my entire education, including college which I didn't finish until I was 60 years old. It was never fun, but something I had to do perfectly. The same way I approached it as a child, trying to squeeze in homework after chores were done.

With regard to school, a child who is having personality problems or the beginning of Mental Disease can either already be experiencing difficulties in school or start having problems. Grades slip, assignments are not done, concentration is impaired, aggressiveness towards other students is frequent, truancy starts, and defying authority begins. Bullying of your child by another student, teacher or administrator can also be the reason for a child's personality changes. As per the Plan of Action, any possible reason for a person's personality change, needs to be explored. It is critical to pay attention to any concerns from teachers, counselors and administrators, with regard to a child's behavior as well as what is happening in school when evaluating problems with a child.

My mother slept a lot. If she wasn't sleeping, she was smoking or talking on the phone to one of her sisters. From what I could hear, it was mostly complaining about my dad. Her animosity toward my dad would continue for as long as I lived with them and beyond. A few times, I told her I thought he worked hard and she got so mad she slapped me across the face. I never defended him again. I made many dangerous cigarette runs for her late at night in a very bad neighborhood. She was very self-centered, mostly worrying if she had enough smokes or nail polish.

She was taking a drug to control her bipolar and other issues. She also had vein problems in her legs and could barely walk as the pregnancy advanced. Eventually, she was in bed all day. I didn't know it at the time but she went off the medications controlling her bipolar when she got pregnant. My dad worked a lot, so my brother, sister and I were on our own most of the time. He had at least two jobs that I knew of. I was always relieved when I heard him open the door late at night after working. I could then fall asleep with my trusty knife under the pillow.

Life was certainly easier for my mother and father and the rest of us with only three children who were very self-sufficient, but my parents obviously didn't have the good judgement to realize that. Considering my mother's mental issues, my father's personality, and the financial situation, they already had all of the children they could reasonably raise. Eighteen months after killing her two little boys, my mother gave birth to her sixth child, followed quickly by her seventh and eighth pregnancies. By the time I was 13, three more children had been added to the family for a total of six. Things got very complicated.

My mother had breakdowns during pregnancy, after giving birth, without being pregnant, during holidays, if the world news was bad, if my father upset her, if something someone said rubbed her the wrong way, and on and on. Her breakdowns were traumatic and involved attempted physical harm to others. Most of the time, we children were alone with her for as much time as it took for my dad to take her to the hospital. She didn't take her medications consistently and marched to her own drum. I had no childhood as on most days I was the mother and she was the child. My goal was to calm her down by saying whatever I thought she wanted to hear, depending on what she was agitated about at that moment. The hope was that she would fall asleep, which she did often. But when she was in a manic state, she could go for days without sleeping. She would take cat naps, but we couldn't trust that she would stay asleep for long and not be up getting into mischief.

My mother had one Electric Shock Treatment (now known as ECT) for sure and maybe more during her first court mandated stay at a psychiatric institution. ECT, known as Electroconvulsive Therapy, sends small electrical currents though the brain triggering a seizure which supposedly eases symptoms of some mental disorders. My mother was found not guilty by reason of insanity and diagnosed as schizophrenic and bipolar. It is still considered very rare to have both disorders together. Today, the disorder is known as Schizoaffective Disorder. The schizophrenia was based on the fact that she repeated over and over to firemen, police and doctors that the devil and other voices in her head told her she needed to get rid of the children to solve her problems, she had hallucinations and delusions, and she also lost total touch with reality.

One of the side effects of ECT, is short term or long term memory loss. I believe my mother might not have remembered anything prior to the day she killed her children. Just as the trauma of watching her kill the boys erased any memories I had of my time on Earth prior to six years old. In any case, my mother was much slower in her thinking when she arrived home, and that never changed. I don't know if my mother was on any specific drugs for schizophrenia when she was released from the hospital or whether they felt the ECT was enough to take care of her demons. For a long time, ECT was a commonly used therapy to rewire circuits in the brain, but is very rarely used in present day. She was on a popular drug for bipolar, which is still the leading drug for this particular mental disorder, but never took it consistently. I do remember that during many of her breakdowns, my mother would be having a conversation with people that definitely weren't in the room.

Because of the stigma of Mental Disease, the patriarch of a certain famous family ordered a lobotomy for his child when he saw signs of mental illness. The procedure went wrong and left the child unable to walk or talk. The child most likely had depression or bipolar and did not require that type of extreme therapy, but in this case the stigma of Mental Disease drove the family to a tragic treatment decision. A lobotomy involved severing connections in the prefrontal cortex of the brain. The last lobotomy was done in 1967 and resulted in the patient's death. The procedure was banned and is no longer performed.

The incidents I remember distinctly when my mother got out of the hospital was talking her through her mini-breakdowns, and there were many. The first time it happened I was scared to death. I had noticed her mental deterioration for a few days. I would come home from school and she was still in her bathrobe. She was complaining about my dad which was typical, and she was walking around from one room to the other. I thought for sure she was going to try to throw me and the other kids out a window, so I started thinking how I was going to defend myself. I would do anything I needed to do to. I hated her. I thought I would kill her if I had to. There were times she definitely had some kind of seizure, although I didn't know what they were at the time. She would shake and her eyes would roll up and down. The frenzy would only last a few minutes, but seemed like an eternity. The scenario was always the same, saying anything I could to agree with her and calm her down, trying desperately to get her to lie down on the bed and hopefully fall asleep, so we could all breathe a sigh of relief. Sometimes it worked, sometimes it didn't.

One incident that put her back in the hospital began because the building was without heat, a frequent occurrence. This time, my mother was already in a fragile state. Before we knew it, she grabbed a butcher knife and started down the stairs to confront the superintendent of the building. I quickly locked the door after she left, glad the knife was not aimed at me, made the two kids hide, and sat down in front of the door. It seemed like an eternity, but soon there was pounding on the door. It was the police. My mother had tried to attack the super with the knife, he prevailed but luckily he did not kill her. My father and uncle got home and an ambulance carted by mother off to a psychiatric hospital. She was gone for a few months that time. Life was always better when she was not home. We eventually got social service help and the women they sent took good care of us. It was much better coming home from school and not worrying about what I would find when I opened the door.

When my mother came home for visits, she complained about everything. Nothing was clean enough, nothing was organized enough, nothing we did was right. She was wrong about it all as we were doing just fine. I continued to think life sucked and just kept getting sadder and sadder. I had no idea we were both fighting Mental Disease, and that it was taking us both down.

A little piece of my mother was gone with each mini and maxi-breakdown and each pregnancy. She was slower, more confused, and smoking two packs or more of cigarettes a day to help keep her calm. She would tell me often she felt like crawling out of her skin she was so nervous. Until I had my first anxiety attack, I didn't understand that feeling. It is horrible and will be discussed in the section on anxiety. Her attention span was non-existent on many days, especially those leading up to a breakdown, and she would spend lots of time staring into space, smoking cigarettes.

I remember my dad, brother, sister and I pulling up to the apartment building after the new baby was born and seeing cop cars all over the place. I know my father thought for sure my mother had killed the new baby. I never saw him move so quickly. It turned out that the owner of the grocery store under the building was stabbed to death. My mother and the baby were safe, except strangely she had left the apartment and he found her up on the roof holding the baby. I can't imagine what he was thinking as he climbed the stairs to the eighth floor and the roof. He never said a word about it, but he never said a word about anything.

My relationship with my father was pathetic. The priest who was very close with my brother, had tickets to see the Ten Commandments. He got sick and couldn't use the tickets and gave them to my mom and dad. My mom didn't feel well and suggested my dad and I go. It was a one hour train trip back and forth to the theater, a half hour walk there and back to the train, and the movie was three hours long. We never said a word to each other the entire time. I was ten and there was so much I wanted to talk about, but not a word came out of my mouth.

My mother never learned to drive. My uncle said she was the worst driver ever and my dad and everyone else gave up trying to teach her. She had no attention span or coordination, and spent the entire time at the wheel smoking and lighting one cigarette after another.

She continued to display other-oriented behavior, hurting others but not herself. She threw a hot iron across the room and barely missed my father, she scratched him many times when he challenged her about not taking her medications, and she slapped me in the face often. It was certainly not abuse, but the reasons for the slaps were not justified. Once she gave me her pink radio as a birthday gift. It was filthy with yellow cigarette smoke and dust and I spent days cleaning it up and enjoying the music until she took it back. I was so upset, I told her she was mean and she slapped me. It reminded me of the slap her mother gave me on the day the boys were killed. I hated both her and my grandmother.

My mother was always saying she could do anything she wanted and that my dad was preventing her from working, traveling and being a star. She honestly believed these things. They were illusions of grandeur and an indication of how out of touch with reality she was. One of her sisters helped her get a job as a cashier at a five and dime. Every night for a week she left the house and went off to work, and every night she came home with a bag of candy or some other treat. In less than a week, she was fired. Her register came up short by a lot of money every night she worked. She tried another job years later at a photo booth. After working for two days, she forgot to lock the door and the entire kiosk was robbed.

There is no doubt that my chronic, stressful childhood made the onset of my own mental illness happen much earlier than it might have if I was raised in a more functional environment. Continuous physical or mental abuse, abandonment, day-to-day fear of living with a mentally ill parent or person, lack of affection and attention, and anxiety with regard to what the future holds can escalate the onset of mental issues and even make them worse if they continue over a long period of time. The Plan of Action will speed up the process of getting help for a child, or any person, as quickly as possible.

From six to twelve years of age, attention needs to be paid to the onset of puberty, which seems to be happening much sooner than it did in the past. The change in hormones and testosterone during this period, can cause sudden personality changes which most of the time are not connected with Mental Disease. On the other hand, puberty can also bring on the beginning of mental illness. Following the Plan of Action will help sort it out. A summary on puberty following this section should also be of assistance.

Another very serious issue that cannot be ignored at any age is misplaced anger which results in physical harm to others, including animals. My mother definitely was what I call other-oriented, doing harm to others. She was not self-destructive and, as a matter of fact, treated herself very well. My aunt said my mother was spoiled and fresh as a child, but I didn't ask specifically if she had anger issues. Anger did manifest itself in her early 20's and was witnessed by relatives who told me about it well after my mother's death. As a matter of fact, weeks before the death of my brothers my mother threw her newborn at my grandmother like he was a football. During that same time, my mother passed the newborn to her neighbor from the same window she threw him out of a few weeks later. The neighbor brought him back, admonishing her for the irresponsible act. Despite two obvious signs that my mother was mentally unstable, the little one was destined to be killed by his mother.

I know many people who admitted doing very ugly things to animals as a child, especially in a group setting, but did not have or develop a mental illness. Close attention must be paid to a child at any age who shows deliberate hostile, physical behavior toward another person or animal. My Plan of Action would recommend an immediate appointment with a physician to rule out any physical problems for the aggression. If the results are negative, then an appointment with a Psychiatrist is the next step. Do not ignore the behavior.

PUBERTY

Puberty is the period when adolescents reach the stage when they can sexually reproduce. The average age for puberty for boys is 12 and the average age for girls is 11, but it can start at any time for either sex. There are many physical changes which are apparent, but there are also mental changes. An adolescent male or female may become confused, emotional, overly sensitive, very angry, lose their temper, and get anxious about their looks and just about everything else. This is the time when distinguishing between puberty and Mental Disease can be frustrating and worrisome.

My mother reached puberty at around 13, according to my aunt, and her mood swings became much more frequent. She started smoking and drinking at 14, and my aunt said that this seemed to settle her down a little. According to her sister, my mother always focused more on the problems of the world than on the everyday issues facing her family. This particular behavior continued throughout her entire life. My aunt reminded me that they lived in a house filled with people who were alcoholics, including their father and all but one of their brothers. Most everyone suffered from depression and all used alcohol and cigarettes to cope. Three of the brothers ended up on skid row, a place where drug addicts and alcoholics congregated.

I didn't reach puberty until I was 16. I had no idea what was happening as it wasn't discussed. I did suffer from increased depression before my period each month. Because hormones can wreak havoc before a period, some people experience disabling mood swings, along with cramping and other physical discomforts. People who have been diagnosed with mental illness sometimes see increased lows during pre-menstruation and while menstruating. Hormones and testosterone play a critical role in physical and mental wellness and when they are out of whack, people can suffer. Most changes in behavior due to puberty are not an indication of mental disorders. On the other hand, any out-of-control chronic behavior in a pubescent needs to be monitored carefully as it could be the beginning of mental health issues

POWER OF ATTORNEY (POA)

I stopped what I was working on in the Guide because of an on-going situation with a family dealing with a mentally ill loved one, which reminded me of the importance of a Power of Attorney. The next section on age includes people over 18, and having legal paperwork in place to help them is paramount. In most states, without this document parents do not have the authority to make healthcare decisions once a child turns 18. It doesn't matter whether the parents are claiming a child as a dependent, paying for health insurance, tuition, life and car insurance, housing, and an allowance, they will be denied access to any medical information if the child is 18 or over. This can be a disaster under any circumstances, but when a child is also mentally ill and doesn't have the clarity or judgement to make decisions about medications and treatments, it can be a life threatening issue. The health care proxy must be signed by the young adult, so it is important to get this done before the person is so out-of-it that they may not agree. Some children (so-called adults) who are not experiencing health or mental issues refuse to sign. There are circumstances where an emergency Power of Attorney can be obtained depending on the circumstances, but it is better to have it in place before the situation is critical.

I would be completely lying if I said the process of determining whether a child is going through a difficult stage in life versus heading toward a Mental Disease diagnosis is simple. It is actually the most complicated, emotional, angst-ridden and frustrating process people face. Imagine having a child who at the age of 14 starts running away, missing school and failing classes, using drugs and alcohol, sleeping too much or not at all, not caring about hygiene, and isolating from the family. It takes a while to figure out what is going on, but the eventual realization is the child needs mental health treatment. A psychiatrist diagnoses depression and anxiety and puts the child on medications. The child is getting talk therapy. A traumatic event is revealed during therapy, and complicates recovery. The child attempts suicide and spends time in a rehab center.

Two years go by and the child is now 16. Every day is spent trying to keep the child on track to take meds regularly, as most people with mental disorders also have an issue with not taking their medications. The goal becomes trying to get the student graduated from high school, a feat requiring tutors and special classes as the child is not well enough to attend school or has been suspended from school. Even on their best days, people who are not stabilized can be disruptive to the entire family. They are generally not the nicest people in the world and are combative, verbally abusive, and sometimes physically abusive, biting, scratching, and hitting family members.

At 18, the child overdoses on an illegal drug, but is saved again. In the hospital, the parents are completely **SHUT OUT OF ANY CRITICAL INFORMATION ON THE CHILD.** Without parents input, the child is COLD TURKEY taken off of a mental health medication prescribed, and sent home. There is one thing that is considered completely irresponsible and that is **taking a patient off of their prescribed meds all at once.** They must be withdrawn gradually, unless there is some kind of life threatening side effect if the med isn't stopped immediately. The parents never get access to the details as to why the child was taken off a drug. Within days, the child attempts suicide again. Because of what they went through, the parents were able to get a Medical Power of Attorney before the third attempt. The child signed it, and is now in a private facility. I expect to get an update on how the private facility worked out for the section on rehabilitation.

This is a true story as are all the examples in this guide and proves why a Power of Attorney is essential when a child has a mental health issue.

The goal of any parent or guardian is to have the child stabilized by 18, but in many cases the years go by and it doesn't happen. There are many different and tragic endings to the example I gave. There are those young adults who give up the constant struggle and use pot and alcohol every day to calm the demons in their brains, living a mostly dysfunctional life. There are the people who leave home, tired of the restrictions and demands of well-meaning family, and end up homeless and often dead in a crack house or dirty alley. Many of these very ill and now deceased people have not agreed to POA's and even have rescinded POA's which were previously in existence.

It is not easy in this day and age to get an 18 year old to sign a Power of Attorney for anything, whether they are mentally healthy or not. Even bribing them with withdrawing support if they don't sign can backfire, as their judgement is way off. They actually think they can survive without support, as they are usually out of touch with reality. Scientists have confirmed that brains aren't fully developed until 25, and there is no doubt about that. To me, it is very simple. As long as parents can prove they are supporting a person who is over 18, they should be able to access medical information for their dependent and make decisions without having to go to court. Unfortunately, there is nothing easy about dealing with mental issues or the legal system in this day and age.

I wish I could give assurances that the process of getting a POA would be easy, but it isn't. All I can suggest is to try to get the paperwork signed during a calm period of mental health when the person you want the signature from is willing to cooperate.

ADOLESCENTS, YOUTHS, YOUNG PEOPLE (TEN TO MID TWENTIES):

The World Health Organization defines adolescents as individuals in the 10 to 19 year age group, youths as 15 to 24 and young people as 10 to 24 years old. Fifteen to 25 is the age group when the diagnosis of Mental Disease happens most frequently, but also the age when diagnosing mental illness is the most challenging. To me, it isn't as important what a certain age group is called as it is to know that the onset of puberty, no matter what age it occurs, is the time when the issues connected with behavioral changes and Mental Disease become blurred and complicated. Without a doubt, the age from puberty (whenever that occurs) to about 25 (when it is believed the brain is fully developed), sees the most frequent manifestations of mental illness. Unfortunately, it is also the most challenging age group to treat. Nowadays, many Psychiatrists and facilities actually decide not to treat people in certain age groups.

It is a shock for many parents to wake up one day and find that a formerly easy-going child has turned into a sullen, rude, demanding, self-centered and emotional mess. A child who once spent hours on hygiene, now won't shower, wash their hair or change clothes. In the majority of cases, this behavior is a direct result of hormonal and testosterone changes which come with puberty. Although families can be thrown into turmoil over a pubescent child, in time with patience, understanding and strict but fair parental guidance, most families come through relatively unscathed.

It is important to know the difference between personality changes due to becoming an adolescent versus behavior which might indicate Mental Disease. I have had experience with my being mentally ill during puberty and adolescence and beyond, living with my mentally ill mother during psychotic and life-threatening breakdowns, and extensive experience with adolescents, both related and not, having mental issues starting with puberty. It is a terrifying time for everyone connected with the people who have a mental illness, and the resources are limited, confusing and filled with frustration. That is why I am hoping the Guide and Plan of Action will help people maneuver through the different aspects of Mental Disease.

My mother had her first psychotic break in her mid-twenties and she killed two innocent people. The adolescent age group continues to be the most dangerous one for suicides, self-harm, attempted murders, mass murders, and nervous breakdowns. When a catastrophe happens and is evaluated, the prognosis in most cases is that the person was showing signs of mental issues for a while beforehand.

Because suicide is the second leading cause of death among 10 to 34-year olds, before I discuss the actual psychological disorders of Mental Disease, this is good time to talk about suicidal ideation. Suicide is a part of many Mental Disease disorders.

SUICIDAL IDIATION

Thinking about taking one's own life and establishing a plan to take one's own life is suicidal ideation. **If there are no plans to commit suicide, but just the thought of wanting to be dead, it is called Passive Suicidal Ideation. When a person is not only thinking about killing themselves but also has a plan for how to do it, and does or does not follow through with that plan, it is known as Active Suicidal Ideation.**

Suicidal thoughts can occur in people without Mental Disease, but it mostly manifests with major depression and the depression found in bipolar disorder. Unfortunately, suicide is on the rise in the United States, and is the second leading cause of death among people from the ages of ten to the mid-thirties.

I personally went through several incidents of passive suicidal ideation during my life, but I never had a concrete plan. As a matter of fact, thinking about the method I would use to kill myself was repulsive to me. Medical researchers believe that there is a malfunction in chemicals in the neurotransmitters in the brain which results in suicidal ideation. There is also the belief that the frontal cortex of the brain lacks adequate blood flow as seen in specific brain scans of many people with suicidal ideation. I was lucky my malfunction did not allow me to go to Active Suicidal Ideation.

There is nothing darker than what a person is feeling when suicide becomes the only way out of a life that has been distorted by a diseased brain. I recently visited a memorial display for Overdose

Awareness Day. As far as the eye could see, there were photos of people who had died of overdoses. This is considered the most popular method of committing suicide for obvious reasons. It's cleaner and easier to collect pills and fill up a glass of water and swallow them, than any other method. For some, there is also the possibility of survival that is generally not the case with hanging, slitting wrists, guns shots to the head, drowning, lying down on a railroad track, and other forms of suicide persons who truly want to be gone choose. I now have a category of suicide I refer to as Suicide by Car. It can be the only explanation for the way people are driving lately. I could not believe the number of beautiful people in these pictures who were no longer with us, because they descended into a darkness so awful and so out of touch with reality that they no longer wanted to be on this earth. **Again, think about the worst day ever in life and how emotionally raw the feelings were and then take that feeling and multiply it a hundred-fold so that reality is a blur and there is no longer any reason to live. Then imagine that continuing day after day after day. This is the plight of a person with suicidal ideation under the umbrella of Mental Disease.**

Sadly, I know about suicide from personal experience. As a matter of fact, I deviated from what I was working on in the guide to do this section because I was informed that someone I knew had been admitted to the hospital because of suicidal ideation. This time it was a passive attempt as it was talked about, but the person did not actually commit the act. The time before was an active suicide attempt, and the person almost died. This person was using prescribed medications for bipolar, but was using pot and other substances to feel better. These substances were interfering with the processing of Mental Disease medications, as well as enhancing the side effects and symptoms. These actions can be deadly, and people are dying this way on a daily basis.

The symptoms to look for which might be a clue to a possible suicide attempt are isolation, talking about death or suicide (although that doesn't always happen), giving stuff away, increased substance use, anger, rage, irritability, mood swings, risky behavior (unprotected sex, out all night, meeting strangers), stealing medication or drugs, saying goodbye inappropriately, and exhibiting extreme anxiety. Some of the above symptoms can be associated with other mental disorders, but talking about death or suicide is something that should never be ignored under any circumstances, especially if the person has attempted suicide in the past. If someone constantly threatens to kill themselves, a serious conversation must take place about the unacceptability of making this threat if it is not true or an attempt to get attention, versus it being a real thought. If it is real, the person needs immediate help and the Plan of Action should be followed.

Regarding Mental Disease, there are people who I describe as other-oriented and people who are self-destructive. The other-oriented person hurts other people, but treats themselves very well. Think mass murderers and people who kill family members or friends. The self-destructive person does harm to themselves and are the most likely to commit suicide. Some engage in slow suicide like cutting themselves, overdosing, drinking into oblivion, not eating properly, participating in risky and life-threatening behavior, not taking their mental health medications, and ignoring their overall health. There are those who are both, of course, and these people are involved in murder-suicide, killing someone and then killing themselves.

Unfortunately, I have experienced all kinds of suicides in my long life, as follows:

A person tragically shoots and kills their spouse and then themselves. Whether there is an indication that a loved one suffers from a mental issue or not, it is never wise to give someone devastating news about the marriage or anything else in an isolated situation, and especially after drinking alcohol. In this case, there was no indication that this person had a mental disorder so severe that they would have been capable of this action. However, a lot of second-guessing goes on after a suicide of any kind and many people suggested that there may have been some indications of depression after all. All too late to prevent the tragedy.

A close relative suffering for years from depression shoots an ex-spouse and then blows their own brains out. Some worried about a possible suicide, but definitely not a murder-suicide.

A friend shoots his wife and then himself, totally stressed due to financial issues caused by his wife's spending habits.

A young person with a supposedly resolved disability issue, beginning a brilliant college career, is found fatally shot by his own hands. The incident is a complete shock to the parents as there was absolutely no indication that there was anything to worry about either physically or mentally. Whatever the person was going through was kept a complete secret, and there were no warnings. This happens frequently, as part of all mental disorders is a devastating tendency to hide feelings.

A young person on a drug with suicidal ideation side effects attempts suicide with a combination of pills and alcohol. There was some talk about not wanting to be alive. The person was using marijuana and alcohol, along with the prescribed medication for depression. This enhanced the suicidal ideation. The person survived the attempt and is currently on several medications for different chemical issues in the brain. Unfortunately, the person is still using pot, etc. to self-soothe. If this continues, there could eventually be dangerous complications.

Another young person recently being treated for anxiety and depression attempts suicide. The attempt was almost successful and the person spent time in the hospital with organ failure issues. There was absolutely no warning of suicide. The person was prescribed one drug after another to resolve the Mental Disease symptoms, but the patient was using pot, alcohol and possibly other illegal drugs to feel better. The mental health medications were being interfered with and could not do their job. This person sounded the alarm recently about suicidal thoughts, and was involuntarily admitted to a hospital for care. They are on three medications for diagnosed imbalances in serotonin, dopamine and other neurotransmitter issues. If this person resumes use of pot, alcohol or illegal drugs, the prognosis for getting the mental disorder under control is very poor. This is happening to thousands of people every single day.

Over the years, I have known people who have committed murder-suicide, attempted suicide, slow suicide, passive suicide and active suicide, and it is a tragedy beyond comprehension. The extent of the dysfunction in the brain for a person to not want to live anymore is as bad as it gets. With help from the drugs developed to stabilize areas of the brain that are not functioning properly, suicidal ideation can be controlled. Illegal drugs, alcohol and marijuana cannot prevent suicide or Mental Disease. As a matter of fact, they enhance the tendency to commit suicide and increase the dysfunction existing in parts of the brain.

What happens when a person attempts suicide? Some suicides are complete shocks, with family and friends not having a clue that the person was thinking about killing themselves. This is a tragedy beyond comprehension for the survivors as they naturally feel guilt for something they really had no control over. They usually need counseling themselves to deal with the repercussions caused by the unexplained death, and to help with the guilt issues.

Most of the time, however, both the suicidal person and family and friends have been through years of dealing with a mentally ill person, following the Plan of Action, and trying to do whatever they can to help solve the crises. To put it frankly, they are exhausted. It doesn't make the attempted suicide any easier to accept, but in many of these cases they are not blindsided and actually are often responsible for saving the person's life more than once.

Most suicides involve taking pills. There are some mentally ill people who are passive about suicide, but sick enough to need the attention that will come with an attempted suicide. They will take just enough to cause alarm and concern, but not enough to kill them. The bottom line is it is a cry for help and they need just as much psychiatric help and rehabilitation as a person who has made a serious attempt at suicide.

If the suicide attempt, regardless of how it is done, results in hospitalization and the person is under 18, parents will have full decision-making and access to medical records during the entire process. That's the good news. The bad news is that the "system" is overloaded. Sometimes beds in mental health facilities are not available and the person has to remain in a bed in a hospital under strict surveillance, as per the law. After the period of time required for surveillance for a suicide attempt has passed, the family has the option to go along with a place where there is a bed available or explore other inpatient or outpatient choices. I am making it sound easier than it is, but it is not. The process of getting a child into a facility is fraught with problems. I will be detailing more of this under the Plan of Action section on Rehabilitation.

If your child is 18, the law identifies them as an "adult" regardless of the fact that they are being fully supported by parents. Under these circumstances, the parent has no right to any information and it is up to the "adult" to keep parents informed or sign a release for them to receive information. A Power of Attorney should be a priority once a mentally ill child turns 18 so that parents can access data relating to their treatment.

Back to the 19-year old who was voluntarily admitted to a hospital for thoughts of taking his life, and the reason why I switched from working on another part of the guide to talking about suicidal ideation. This person made a sincere attempt at suicide with an overdose of pills a year earlier. After being in critical care for days with a damaged liver and kidneys, the person went to rehab and came out with a diagnosis of bipolar disease and anxiety disorder. I said I would not reveal any drug treatments in this guide as only a Psychiatrist has that ability. I do not have the credentials to mention actual drugs used for treatment, even though my experience has given me much knowledge on mental health medications. This is what Psychiatrists train many long and hard years to do, and it is a challenge of monumental proportions especially these days with so many drugs available. Unfortunately, because most people do not get a brain scan for a conclusive determination of where the imbalances in their brain are, very rarely do they respond to the first drugs prescribed for them. Blood tests are not the most effective way to determine what the level of serotonin, dopamine or other chemicals are and so sometimes a prescription is hit or miss. Blood work also cannot assess what the health is of the neurons and the millions of other circuits in the brain. Sometimes, boosters need to be added to the original medication. Every patient is different and what works for one may not work for another, even though they have the same disorder.

After being treated and released from the suicide attempt, this person went back to using pot and alcohol to help cover up the demons in the brain. The mental illness drugs prescribed did not even have time to have an impact on the brain before the pot and alcohol inhibited the effectiveness of the meds. There was never any success with the drugs prescribed for the mental disorder. **I have said before I firmly believe that a person with Mental Disease will never see any improvement as long as they use pot, heroin, any other illegal drugs and alcohol to help them feel better.**

If there is also addiction disorders in the family, life-threatening health issues, and serious mental disorders, complete dysfunction can result. Many people end up homeless in these situations because support from family and friends stops, mainly because the person disrupts the home by stealing, bringing home other drug addicts, alcoholics and mentally ill people, and physically abusing family members. There are millions of people living in fear of their own loved ones.

The saga of the 19 year old continues. The second admittance to a hospital for a passive suicide attempt was voluntary. In the dead of night, the patient was transferred to a facility out-of-state. Because the parents did not have a POA, which is needed when a "child" is over 18 and considered an "adult" they could not get any information. To add insult to injury, because of the pandemic they could not even visit their child. They had no idea what treatment was being done. During the time at the second facility, the patient was withdrawn "cold turkey" from a medication he was taking. **NO MENTAL HEALTH PROFESSIONAL WILL EVER CONDONE REMOVING A MENTALLY ILL PERSON FROM A DRUG COLD TURKEY,** unless there is a life threatening reaction to the medication. There is even a name associated with this called Antidepressant Withdrawal Syndrome (ADS).

The 19-year old patient was released, and a few days later had a severe psychotic break, attempting active (thought about, planned and acted on) suicide with a weapon. After mom and dad tried for a long time to get the weapon dropped, a policeman was able to say just the right thing: "you are not the only one who feels life is not worth living and are in pain, we police feel it all day, every day". The weapon was finally dropped. The person was taken by ambulance to the hospital and is now undergoing another effort to get the right medications to resolve the brain malfunction. This time, the patient was given an antipsychotic drug because of signs of psychosis that were part of the diagnosis.

There is nothing more physically and mentally exhausting than living with a mentally ill person, especially when they are not responding to treatment. The constant day-to-day vigilance trying to keep them from going over the edge, doing harm to themselves or others, causing disturbances with other family members, keeping up with therapy appointments and doctor's visits, monitoring medicines, and reaching out for help can bring down the strongest of people. A strong support system is critical.

The figures on suicide are convoluted by the fact that many people commit suicide by overdosing on drugs. Depending on the circumstances surrounding the event, a suicide could be misconstrued as an overdose. When the person does not survive an overdose, it is difficult to ascertain what their intentions were. Because of

70

the stigma of suicide and Mental Disease in general, family members may not divulge that the person was suicidal. They may not have even known that their loved one was thinking about taking their life. Most overdoses are not attempts at suicide, but unfortunately the drugs kids are taking nowadays are laced with other deadly drugs.

The following represents the final discussion regarding Mental Disease in particular age groups. It focuses on adults and seniors, and suicidal ideation is also common in this group as they face challenging aging issues.

ADULTS/SENIORS:

Mental health disorders are the leading cause of disability in adults in the United States. An estimated 40 million adults suffer from some form of mental health issue, with anxiety at the top of the list. Six million are known to have bipolar disorder and the numbers are climbing rapidly.

The goal nowadays is to try to help a person become functional with Mental Disease as soon as possible. Unfortunately, many people do not have the resources or the will to get help. There are many reasons why people find themselves still suffering from Mental Disease well into maturity. I was 60 before I sought help. Growing up in the 1950's and 1960's meant keeping quiet about feeling depressed because it was a definite stigma. Unfortunately, this is still the case. Another reason for not getting help is poor judgement in thinking and believing it is normal to feel rotten about life all the time. It was a clinical trial that I did not end up qualifying for which allowed me to live a demon-free life for 14 good years on a medication that has worked for me. I will never forget the day, the time, and where I was when the concrete block I carried around from the time I was 6 years old, disappeared from my shoulders. I thank my wonderful

Psychiatrist and Psychiatric Nurse every day for what they did for me.

I WILL SAY THIS AGAIN, ONE OF THE BIGGEST DETRIMENTS TO A PERSON BEING ABLE TO LIVE A FUNCTIONAL LIFE WITH MENTAL DISEASE IS THE FACT THAT THEY HAVE CHOSEN DRUGS AND/OR ALCOHOL AS A 'FIX' FOR THEIR MENTAL DISORDER. Some people never got the benefit of proper treatment due to lack of insurance, money, family support, outright rejection of any treatment, and turning to pot and other illegal drugs to self-soothe. In most cases, it is easier to use drugs and drink because they have no other choice. Before they know it, they are in their 30's, 40's and older, homeless or living in crack houses. THERE IS NO DOUBT IN MY MIND THAT MENTAL DISEASE AND ADDICTION DISORDERS GO HAND IN HAND.

There are many sad stories of mentally healthy adults suddenly suffering from early onset Dementia (Alzheimer's and Senility are common parts of this disorder), Lewy Body Dementia, Depression and other related disorders. These disorders are also caused by chemical irregularities in the brain that are present in cases of Mental Disease seen in all age groups. They manifest with the same symptoms as Mental Disease in many cases and can co-exist with psychotic conditions. Dementia does impact mental health, but many experts don't identify it as a Mental Disease. The main symptoms for Dementia is memory struggles and the inability to communicate. But it is not that simple, because symptoms of Mental Disease disorders are also seen in some people with Dementia. The treatment is similar to that for a mental disorder, because Dementia involves the same chemical neurotransmitters that are defective in the brain. It involves too little or too much serotonin or dopamine and many areas of Ischemic strokes damaging the billions of neurons in the average brain, and all needing to be neutralized by medications developed to help those damaged areas.

Depression is the most common mental disorder in adults (seniors). It is also a main symptom of Dementia. It is well-known and documented that seniors left alone for long periods of time suffer more depression than those who are not socially isolated. Sometimes an anti-depressant will help if depression is the only symptom. Changing the environment to one with more social interaction should also be a priority.

Age is the main factor in determining whether a person has a Mental Disease or Dementia symptoms. If the symptoms are mainly a loss of memory, confusion, an extreme personality change, and inability to communicate with no other issues, it is generally diagnosed as Dementia. However, dementia can also manifest with hallucinations, paranoia, agitation, delusions, and manic behavior. There are occasions of late-onset schizophrenia and late onset bipolar in adults, but because there are symptoms of hallucinations and paranoia, mania, agitation, and delusions connected with dementia, it can be very complicated to diagnose.

An adult who has battled Mental Disease all of their lives tends to die sooner due to illnesses and injuries related to their struggles.

My mother died at 50 of cancer, her immune system broken by years of chain smoking, Electroshock treatments, 10 pregnancies, weight issues and poor nutrition, misuse of mental health drugs, and constant nervous breakdowns and hospitalizations. Many adults have passed away from gunshots, beatings and other injuries directly related to the need to support their lifestyle by stealing drugs, alcohol and money. Many have committed slow suicide with dirty needles and drugs resulting in liver and kidney damage. They pass of diseases related to trading sex for drugs and alcohol and even a temporary roof over their heads. Some have died of full body organ shutdown as their loved ones sit by their beds for days and weeks. Sometimes, the hope is for a quick passing as the person has suffered and caused suffering for years with their inability to conquer their demons. I have seen and heard it all, and written more condolence cards than I can begin to count. Many times, there is relief for the surviving family after years of stress and sadness. *They are at peace* is a statement that definitely is true for the deceased mentally ill person.

I am sorry to say that overall our success in getting adults with Dementia stabilized is just as complicated, confusing and difficult as the success with other age groups suffering with Mental Disease. The system is **OVERWHELMED** with cases of people inflicted with brain diseases and there are simply not enough facilities and specialists available to cope with the magnitude of the situation. I may have said this before and might say it again but my fantasy is to win the lottery big time and open up a free clinic offering SPECT scans of the brain with diagnosis and prescriptions for medications to treat the areas that are defective. I truly believe that just like cancer, mental illness is a disease that needs to be diagnosed with brain scans and proper medications before the person can do any talk therapy that would benefit them. A person who has a mastectomy wouldn't start therapy to strengthen the arms before the mastectomy. The same goes for Mental Disease. I know for a fact, because I lived through it, that it is a waste of time to do group counseling, talk therapy, or any other program **UNTIL THE MENTALLY ILL PERSON IS ON A MEDICATION THAT HAS STABILIZED THEM ENOUGH SO THAT THEY CAN UNDERSTAND AND BENEFIT FROM THE**

NEXT STEP. For example, they don't give speech therapy to people before they have brain surgery that might result in loss of speech.

The need is to place Mental Disease in the same category as other diseases and treat the obvious physical disease of the brain. The new SPECT exam should be considered seriously for diagnosing brain issues. Unfortunately, as has happened initially with so many other machines which have been developed, it is not covered by health insurance and is not considered seriously by the mental health community. Same old, same old. It might make diagnosis of mental illness easier, and that scares some people for monetary reasons.

I remember when the only thing available for colon cancer was a torturous procedure known as sigmoidoscopy, which only covered half the colon, resulting in many colon cancer deaths. Just think of a stiff pipe up your butt probing the lower portion of your bowel with no anesthesia. The worst pain I have ever felt in my life, and I was forced back for more torture. Sadly, I had polyps in the upper areas of my colon which were never seen by this incompetent procedure. It took too long for the colonoscopy, under anesthesia to become the only treatment recommended to cover the entire colon, thus reducing colon cancer deaths dramatically.

I consider the SPECT to be the current best diagnosis for Mental Disease, and I hope and pray that it won't be long before it is considered in the same vein as the colonoscopy. Cure the brain and then the person can respond to behavioral therapy treatments as needed. Recently, Dr. Phil of the long-standing television show, reiterated this same point by saying, you can't do talk therapy with a mentally ill person until the brain has been examined and the proper medications administered to correct the chemical imbalances.

This type of brain scan would also make it easier and quicker to diagnose our senior population and prescribe medications which would help those areas of their brains that are deteriorating. This could stop the progress of the disease and give them more time to enjoy family and friends. If the meds can stop them from "sundowning" (becoming very agitated and unstable usually after the sun goes down), it can delay them from having to enter a nursing facility and leaving their families.

After I established my Living with Mental Disease group on Facebook, I was asked multiple times to include in the Guide a list of things that would indicate a cause for concern with a senior living independently.

1. ADL'S = sitting, standing, walking, bathing and grooming on their own.

2. Physical appearance – sudden loss or gain of weight, bruising, dark circles or bags under the eyes, not looking clean or well-rested. Evidence they are not taking prescription drugs regularly.

3. Home – the environment should be sanitary and uncluttered for safety reasons.

4. Social – should be making and answering calls, should not be deliberately isolating, should be enjoying favorite hobbies, should know exactly what to do in case of an emergency, and should know what is available in their community.

5. Mental – should be using good judgement with regard to their limitations, should not have trouble communicating,

should be close to the same personality as they had through life, should not be exhibiting concerning mood swings, should not be abusing themselves or others, and should not be obsessively talking about suicide.

PSYCHOLOGICAL DISORDERS/SYNDROMES

The following is a list of psychological disorders/syndromes which manifest themselves from puberty to adulthood. They are rarely seen in infants and toddlers, but cannot be totally ruled out for any age when personality changes warrant diagnosis and attention to the Plan of Action. I am focusing on disorders I have had experience with, but there are many others out there and would take more than this Guide to address all of them.

General Anxiety/Panic Attacks and Anxiety Disorder:
General Anxiety is considered the most common mental concern in the United States at this time. Interestingly, occasional anxiety at the right level can keep people more alert and focused. Unfortunately, when anxiety is out of control it can include shortness of breath, heart palpitations, sweating and dry mouth. It is a frequent occurrence in this day and age and especially during puberty. External issues like worrying about looks, stressful schedules, popularity, school, using illegal drugs and alcohol, and family dynamics can make the anxiety worse.

Communicating about issues and relieving stressful situations can ease anxiety in many cases. Children have a lot of expectations to meet these days and that in itself can cause anxiety. Sometimes the thyroid acts up during this period of time, and it is worth it to have a test done if the anxiety is frequent and severe despite attempts to alleviate it with behavioral changes.

I had anxiety as a child, but it was very physical with bowel problems and nausea. I didn't know until I was in my mid-20's that I had a diseased gallbladder (yes, a person can be born with a non-functional gallbladder that causes havoc until it is removed). I was always afraid and worried about everything and overwhelmed every day. I thank goodness the anxiety was mild and that I was able to function to help my parents with an ever-growing family. Keep in mind, with general anxiety the person is **FUNCTIONAL**.

Anxiety Disorder happens when feelings of distress and fear are so overwhelming in situations that are not threatening that **the person cannot function.** Symptoms are the same as for anxiety, but are more severe and frequent. Anxiety Disorder can exist by itself, but depression almost always includes anxiety disorder. The Plan of Action calls for an appointment with a Psychiatrist because with Anxiety Disorder, the person is generally **NOT FUNCTIONAL**.

Panic disorder, obsessive-compulsive disorder, and phobias are included under Anxiety Disorder and if severe can result in a person not being able to function.

I had General Anxiety on many occasions during my life, but I have never experienced anxiety to the point where I could not function. I definitely have been around many people with anxiety, both functional and dysfunctional. With my general anxiety, I had heart palpitations and some difficulty accomplishing tasks, but I have seen people who complained that their heart felt like it was coming out of their chest, that couldn't accomplish any task, and would literally walk around in circles all day. Some ended up going into a full-blown panic attack.

One case involved a 14-year old with depression, who also had symptoms of Anxiety Disorder. The adolescent suffered years of feeling overwhelmed, paranoid, exhausted, angry, sad, manic, involved in risky behavior such as running away, not going to school, using drugs and alcohol, not caring about hygiene or appearance, failing classes, and isolating from family. There was a trauma which definitely complicated behavior, but there was also history of Mental Disease on both sides of the family. The teen was getting as much help as possible and was on anti-depressants and anti-anxiety medications, but eventually made a serious attempt at suicide with pills and alcohol. The teen was extremely upset when revived and was admitted for psychiatric care with a diagnosis of bipolar, including anxiety disorder. There may have been some medicines the teen was taking to help anxiety and depression which may have helped cause the suicidal ideation, or not. When a person is taking medications, it is important to know what the side effects might be and to remain cognizant of changes in behavior which might foretell of serious problems. In any case, during this crisis the person was not considered FUNCTIONAL on most days and did warn of a possible suicide attempt.

The second experience involved a 17 year old, who was perfect in everything as a child including sports, school, personality, and behavior. The adolescent was extremely busy and in high school started experiencing anxiety, but didn't mention it at all. Instead, kept pushing through an extremely rigorous schedule of school and athletic functions. This might have been a case of General Anxiety becoming Anxiety Disorder. The person is able to function initially (general anxiety), but eventually by the time they are in high school or college, cannot function (anxiety disorder). What initially started out as occasional feelings of being overwhelmed, sweating, dry mouth, heart palpitations, poor judgement, confusion, an inability to say no, afraid to fail, worrying about what people thought and were saying, eventually became a full-blown Anxiety Disorder where the person COULD NOT pay attention to anything because of the obsessive magnitude of the anxiety symptoms. A major breakdown occurred. In this case, there was also a failed attempt at suicide with pills. The eventual prognosis was bipolar and anxiety disorder. A combination of long-term stress and a family history of Mental Disease also contributed to this outcome.

Another more recent case involves a young man who has serious anxiety, but refuses to use the drug prescribed for anxiety disorder. After only three days on it, the person decided the medicine made him sleepy and so quit taking it. This happens in many cases where the patient does not give the medicine a chance to work, complaining about side effects which would most likely disappear after time on the drug. In other situations the effects of the drug have to be weighed against the issues going on with the mental disorder. In this case, a feeling of tiredness was a small price to pay for the extreme anxiety the young person was dealing with on a frequent basis. The person was already exhibiting very serious physical symptoms from the anxiety including heart palpitations and shortness of breath, which will get worse without medication. The outcome will not be positive for quality of life without medication to control the chronic anxiety.

Again, another reminder to investigate your family history, both physically and mentally, as it may help save a life someday. It is paramount not to ignore personality changes in anyone at any age, especially if there is Mental Disease in the family.

Please download surveys for anxiety, depression, bipolar, suicidal ideation, etc. They can help define symptoms of mental disorders and even determine the seriousness of these symptoms. I have found them very helpful and they are also used by mental health professionals to assess patients. I believe the more a person knows about what is going on, the better they can cope with the situation and get the right help.

Remember that people with anxiety, depression, etc., tend to cover up pain with alcohol and drugs. Unfortunately, if they have also inherited addiction disorders, this can cause major complications for treatment. It is unacceptable to combine alcohol, drugs and prescriptions for mental disorders. The prescriptions are rendered useless and the drugs and alcohol only provide a temporary solution to a long-term problem.

Major Depressive Disorder (MDD):

Think about the worst day ever in life and imagine feeling that way every day. Now imagine that does not even come close to what a person who is depressed is going through. I have often said I wish everyone could walk in the shoes of someone who is depressed for just one day in order to get a true understanding of what it is like. So many people think it is an easy thing to control, but that is not true. MDD really has nothing to do with a person's lifestyle. They could appear to be the most successful and happy people in the world (think Robin Williams, renowned comedian, suffering lifelong depression resulting in suicide) and yet they are fighting despondency, sleep disorders, fatigue, eating issues, loss of interest, memory problems, inability to make decisions, worry, social withdrawal, anxiety, self-harm, addiction to drugs and alcohol, and thoughts of suicide. Daily tasks and relationships can be very difficult to maintain. It can be a one-time occurrence (very rare) or last a lifetime.

Persistent Depressive Disorder (PDD):

The symptoms are very similar for both PDD and MDD, but the experts say they are not as intense with PDD. PDD lasts for two years or longer, but MDD can also last for a lifetime. Daily functioning with PDD is considered easier than with MDD. It is the most common type of depression, and the severity of symptoms can fluctuate. Some people believe that feeling the way they do is a normal part of life.

Persistent Depressive Disorder represents the kind of depression I suffered from my entire life until I was diagnosed at 60 years old, and put on an anti-depressant. I will never forget as long as I live when the medicine kicked in about three days after being prescribed, and I looked up at the bright blue sky and said, "is this the way normal people feel?". It was like a black cloud had been smothering me all of my life and suddenly lifted. I still had to work on days to kick the demons out of my brain, but not in any way close to the kind of horror I went through trying to function and survive prior to the anti-depressant. This disease made it hard for me to find any joy in my life despite all the good things that were happening. I was glad to be rid of it.

Bipolar Disorder (Manic Depression):

Manic Depression is the former name for Bipolar Disorder. It manifests in abnormally high and low mood swing. A person can feel very excited or energetic and at other times sink into depression. These mood swings can last for days, weeks or months. The highs are manic episodes and the lows are depressive episodes.

The two types of Bipolar Disorder are Bipolar 1 and Bipolar 2. The difference between 1 and 2 is in the severity of the manic episodes. The manic episodes with Bipolar 1 are more severe, and may require hospitalization. A person suffering from Bipolar 1 may never have a major depressive episode, while a person with Bipolar 2 will definitely experience depressive issues.

In order to be diagnosed with Bipolar 1 Disorder, at least one episode of mania must be involved. Manic symptoms include high energy, racing thoughts and speech, irritability, lack of sleep, feelings of grandeur, participating in risky and/or destructive behavior, feeling elated, increased confidence and self-esteem. The depression part of this disorder has the same symptoms as Major Depressive Disorder (tiredness, irritability, trouble concentrating, lack of interest in anything, etc.). When severe, there may be hallucinations and delusions. Mania and depression symptoms can be separate or mixed. Changing moods can be rapid, intense and confusing. During a manic episode, there is no doubt that something is very wrong. The word Hypomania is also worth talking about. This is a manic episode which is less severe than a full-blown manic episode. Hypomania can occur in people who are under the influence of drugs or alcohol.

Bipolar does have a hereditary component and so the risk of getting it is higher if a parent or sibling have it.

The following is one of the best personal accounts of having Bipolar I have read from a person who was brave enough to ignore the stigma and admit she has a Mental Disease:

"There is nothing I don't know about my Bipolar 1 disorder. I was on again, off again with my medications for years. There is a reason for this, it's called Anosognosia, which means lack of insight. When we start to feel better, we don't believe we are sick so why take our medication. Our brains are playing a trick on us. Anosognosia is what makes treating Bipolar so difficult. There is a go-to medication that has actually worked for Bipolar Disorder since the 1950's and before, and it is also considered to help prevent suicide. We have a high suicide rate, 1 in 3. General population rate is 1 in 30. It has been proven that Lithium is the anti-suicide medication. When we are manic, we make horrible decisions due to the inability to understand the consequences. When we are depressed, we attempt suicide. Our life is a roller coaster ride from hell. Although on medications, an episode can be triggered by lack of sleep, stress, death in the family, or really anything".

I value the opinions of people who are suffering with Mental Disease as it helps other people to understand what might be happening to them. Their experiences are invaluable and totally ignored in the quest to improve the serious issues connected with Mental Disease. That has to change!

Again, as per the Plan of Action, physical exams and thyroid tests must be performed because many symptoms of hypothyroidism are similar to depressive symptoms or mood disorders. If everything is negative, a mental health professional will investigate all symptoms to make a diagnosis. Even at that, it is never easy to diagnose a mental disorder. Unfortunately, brain scans are still not considered the first line of defense in diagnosing Mental Disease and that also has to change. In reality, what Psychiatrists are doing nowadays is giving multiple choice tests, examining distinct symptoms and behavior, talking to the patient and caretakers, and taking blood work. It is a long and complicated process, which could be made easier and quicker with brain scans.

Schizoaffective Disorder:
This disorder is a combination of three disorders under the umbrella of Mental Disease. They are Schizophrenia, Bipolar, and Depression. Bipolar Type and Depressive Type are the two types of Schizoaffective Disorder. The psychotic symptoms vary from one person to another, but usually include hallucinations, delusions, impaired communication and speech, bizarre behavior, symptoms of depression (sad) insomnia, manic mood, impaired functioning, and problems with

personal hygiene. The mood disorders can be either bipolar type which would include mania and sometimes depression, or depressive type. For diagnosis, a major depressed or manic mood episode and at least a two-week period of psychotic symptoms (without a major mood episode) must have occurred.

My mother was found "not guilty by reason of insanity" by a Court of Law in 1953 for killing my two baby brothers. She was admitted to a mental institution where she was diagnosed with Bipolar and Schizophrenia, a very unusual situation at that time to see both disorders diagnosed together. The Schizophrenia was based on the voices she said she heard which told her she had to get rid of all of her children, and of course her symptoms of depression. She told everyone who made contact with her on that day about the voices, and definitely the doctors at the mental institution where she ended up. These voices were considered hallucinations. She received one Electric Shock Treatment (possibly two or more, but never confirmed), and released in less than a year. Whether the EST treatment knocked out her memory of the boys and the event or she chose to forget about them remains a question mark. No one had the nerve to bring it up. She was too fragile, and she never talked about the boys for the rest of her life.

It takes poor judgement on the part of parents to honestly believe they can properly raise ten children, especially when one of the parents is chronically mentally ill. My mother was seriously ill with illusions of grandeur, hallucinations, delusions, dangerous risky behavior aimed at others, and all of the other symptoms of Bipolar and Schizophrenia. It was a recipe for disaster as she continued to get pregnant, giving birth to five more children after being released from the mental institution. She continued to be dictated by voices telling her what she should do during her nervous breakdowns, which were frequent. She was self-centered and it was always about her well-being. Some Bipolar and Schizophrenia results in self-destructive behavior and/or harming others. With my mother, the destruction was aimed at her children and to an extent my father, but he was big enough to defend himself.

While she took her medication for the Bipolar issue (I believe she was prescribed nothing for the Schizophrenia as it was believed it was resolved with Electroshock Treatments), she was just functional enough to take care of her family. Unfortunately, with most mental disorders, and especially Bipolar, **the patient stops taking the medication once they start feeling better**. It is called Anosognosia. It is actually a big part of the disease, which is very concerning. I remember my father struggling with my mother to get pills in her mouth. She would throw things at him and hit him to avoid taking her medication. More often than not, he would give up and go to work. And then the mania and depressive episodes (she had both) would begin, lasting for weeks.

It was frightening dealing with a person in the throes of a Bipolar/Schizophrenic breakdown, whether I was 8, 10, 12, 15 or 17. The mania was almost worse than the depressive state. During manic episodes, she was convinced she could do anything. She NEVER slept. It would take an entire book to detail all of the manic events, but on one occasion all six of us kids ended up being piled into a taxi cab to a store with the promise of seeing Santa. She ended up getting into an argument with the taxi cab driver after smoking in his cab and spitting on the floor. She refused to pay him and he called the police. We did get into the store, but she caused a ruckus with Santa and my father was called to come rescue us.

When we went to family events, she would always end up getting mad and walking out, often late at night, with one or more of us kids in tow. We never knew where we were going. It was reckless and risky walking through dark streets, with her ranting and raving about how bad the people in the family were. In reality, it was all in her sick mind as they had done nothing. Other issues were leaving the house naked, running away from people coming to pick her up to take her to the hospital, hiding from my father so he couldn't take her away when he finally realized she couldn't stay at home, concocting plans to get a cab and travel a long distance to see someone, and talking on the phone for hours to relatives in another state, complaining about us kids and my dad. She would walk around in circles for hours, pacing back and forth, agitated about everything. Her eyes were that of an alien.

Depressive episodes were also very scary. We had to worry about her intentions to hurt others. She did put one of the babies out in the snow, poured milk down the throat of another, had no interest in taking care of the children, went after one with a knife, threw hot coffee several times at myself and my father, destroyed personal property belonging to others, stole money, and generally wreaked havoc during all of her waking hours. The object was to get her to stay in bed and sleep to protect ourselves, but her sleeping habits were way off. My nerves were on edge every minute of the day. I have never since talked so much bull crap to one person as I did to my mother to calm her down. I would say whatever I needed to say to convince her that she was the greatest person in the world and that she had a right to feel the way she did. It was the only thing that worked, and sometimes that didn't calm her down. It was exhausting.

WHEN IN THE PRESENCE OF A MENTALLY ILL PERSON IN THE THROES OF A NERVOUS BREAKDOWN, NEVER AGITATE THEM. Whatever it takes to keep them calm, do it until help arrives and you are no longer alone. If the person is threatening harm to themselves or others, or seems to be suicidal, call 911 immediately.

As I have said, I don't know if the fact that I had to stay functional to protect my life and the life of others helped me to cope with my own hopelessness and sadness. As they say, people with Persistent Depressive Syndrome sometimes believe that what they are feeling is just a part of normal life. That definitely became me. I often wonder if people who don't have obstacles in their lives, succumb more to the symptoms of Mental Disease because they have not had to struggle in order to survive. It is something I would love to research. I am thankful every day that I did not inherit the devastating mental disorders my mother and so many of her family members were born with.

I don't know if my mother would have fared better if she had been made to face the death of her children. I certainly think it would have helped. Even with medication that works, I do believe that a mentally ill person cannot truly heal unless they face their demons, and that is what we hope happens when Psychiatrists, Psychologists, and Therapists are working together.

IT IS NEVER ACCEPTABLE TO USE ALCOHOL AND DRUGS WHEN TAKING MEDICATIONS FOR MENTAL DISEASE. Also, severe stress, use of drugs, alcohol abuse, and trauma (past or present including childhood abuse or death of a loved one) can trigger Bipolar, Schizophrenic, and Schizoaffective Disorders.

EATING DISORDERS

EATING DISORDERS involve disruptive eating patterns and obsessive concerns about weight which impact physical and mental health. Eating disorders can be diagnosed in infancy and early childhood, especially with Autism. Anorexia Nervosa is described as a fear of gaining weight and a very distorted and unrealistic view of appearance and behavior. The person restricts food consumption leading to dangerous and sometimes deadly weight loss and low body weight. Bulimia Nervosa involves a person binging on food and then vomiting, using laxatives or diuretic, and exercising excessively to compensate for the binging. Rumination Disorder is seen in people who are developmentally or intellectually delayed. The person regurgitates their food in order to spit it out or swallow it again. Pica involves craving and consuming non-food substances such as dirt, paint or soap. It is commonly associated with children who have developmental disabilities. I must admit that I started eating dirt from the sides of buildings and underneath car wheel wells when I was reunited with my family. It lasted a couple of years. I was never diagnosed with developmental disabilities, but I discovered during research on the issue that Pica can also occur when a person is very low on iron. I assume that was the case with me. A new disorder, Binge-Eating Disorder, has been added to this group. The individual consumes large amounts of food over a couple of hours for which they feel they have no control over. The episodes are usually triggered by boredom, stress, anxiety or extreme euphoria.

PERSONALITY DISORDERS

PERSONALITY DISORDERS are chronic maladaptive patterns of thoughts, feelings, and behaviors which result in serious relationship problems and detriments to most areas of life. Many people have said personality disorders are the worst of all the mental disorders. I am not sure, as I believe they are all devastating.

Antisocial Personality Disorder

I do feel that *Antisocial Personality Disorder* is the worst of the Personality Disorders because it includes the dangerous Psychopaths and Sociopaths. Antisocial Personality Disorder is described as people who disregard rules, social norms and the rights of others (known as *Sociopaths)*. Symptoms can start in childhood and manifest in a lack of empathy for others and a lack of remorse after destructive behavior. This disorder also includes *Psychopaths* who have the same issues as *Sociopaths,* except their social behavior is much more abnormal and violent with criminal tendencies. Many mass murderers have been diagnosed with Antisocial Personality Disorder.

Recently, a person killed multiple people blaming his actions on sexual addiction. He claimed that in order to get rid of the horrible way he was feeling, he had to eliminate the temptations. His sexual addiction personality disorder combined with Antisocial Personality Disorder resulted in a mass murderer. A panel of Psychiatrists will test for an official diagnosis to determine if he is mentally ill. In this case, a SPECT exam would be a valuable tool in determining how his brain compares to a normal brain.

Avoidant Personality Disorder

Avoidant Personality Disorder manifests in feelings of insecurity so severe that social inhibition and rejection sensitivity prevent the individual from functioning in daily life.

Borderline Personality Disorder

Borderline Personality Disorder manifests in impulsive actions, unstable interpersonal relationships and self-image, and severe emotional instability.

Narcissistic Personality Disorder

Narcissistic Personality Disorder is a self-centered disorder, where the person is only concerned for themselves. They have a completely exaggerated positive self-image, are totally self-centered and have low or no empathy for others. Having no empathy for others can be very dangerous if the person is a caretaker of another human being. I am afraid that our present culture might be producing more narcissists, with people needing more attention and having a distorted sense of their self-worth. It is one thing to have self-esteem, but it is another thing to have a totally unrealistic view of accomplishments.

Obsessive-Compulsive Personality Disorder

Obsessive-Compulsive Personality Disorder manifests in a chronic pattern of preoccupation with orderliness, perfection, inflexibility and mental and interpersonal control. People with this disorder suffer from obsessive thoughts about many things including hurting themselves or others. I have known several people with this disorder and they were miserable people, because the thoughts never stopped until they were medicated. This is a different condition than obsessive compulsive disorder (OCD), where the individual obsesses with repetitive motions such as washing hands every few minutes.

Paranoid Personality Disorder

Paranoid Personality Disorder is characterized by a distrust of others whether they are family or friends. There doesn't need to be justification or evidence of bad intentions for the distrust to be perceived.

Histrionic Personality Disorder

Histrionic Personality Disorder is connected with attention-seeking behavior. The person will do just about anything to attract attention away from others and onto themselves, even if the behavior is inappropriate.

Schizoid Personality Disorder

Schizoid Personality Disorder manifests in social detachment. These people are indifferent to relationships, concerned more about their own lives, and appear cold and aloof without emotional expression.

Schizotypal Personality Disorder

Schizotypal Personality Disorder is similar to Schizoid Personality Disorder, except the person has definite speech, appearance, behavior, and thought eccentricities.

Unfortunately, there are many other personality disorders and too many for me to detail in this guide. I have not had experience with all of the disorders, but I have come in contact with individuals suffering from all of the above during my lifetime.

POST TRAUMATIC STRESS DISORDER (PTSD)

POST TRAUMATIC STRESS DISORDER (PTSD) usually develops when a person has experienced exposure to violence (sexual or otherwise), serious injury, or exposure to actual or threatened death. Symptoms include avoidance of anything which reminds the individual of the event, reliving the event, having constant negative thoughts, being on edge, having nightmares, flashbacks, bursts of anger, and concentration problems. Regarding serious injury such as constant concussions suffered by athletes or people in combat, I believe brain scans are absolutely necessary to diagnose the areas of the brain which might be damaged. I am not buying the thought that only an autopsy of the brain can tell us what was going on with the afflicted person. I am still researching the brain scan issue.

PSYCHOLOGICAL (PSYCHIATRIC) DISORDERS

PSYCHOLOGICAL (PSYCHIATRIC) DISORDERS are patterns of behavior that create distress in many areas of a person's life. This category includes **Neurodevelopmental Disorders**, which are usually diagnosed during infancy, childhood or adolescence. An example of a Neurodevelopmental Disorder is *Intellectual Disability* (formerly known as mental retardation), which is typically diagnosed before the age of 18. It also includes *Global Developmental Delay*, which are developmental disabilities in cognition, social functioning, motor skills, language and speech under the age of five. This can be a temporary diagnosis until the child is able to take an IQ test when they are older.

Communication Disorder is included in this group and impacts the ability to understand and use language and speech.

Autism Spectrum Disorder is also a part of this area of mental disorders. It consists of repetitive and restricted behavior patterns and chronic deficits in social interaction and communication in many areas of life. These symptoms are usually present very early in life and cause serious impairment in occupational and social functioning. People with Autism are also impacted by the change of seasons and Daylight Savings Time (see section on SAD below).

Attention-Deficit Hyperactivity Disorder (ADHD) is included in this group of disorders. Symptoms are lack of attention, hyperactive behavior, and poor impulse control which interferes with several areas of life (social, home, school, work, etc.).

There are so many other disorders in this category that should be discussed like SAD, *Seasonal Affective Disorder,* in which the person experiences depression during certain times of the year. I was depressed all the time, but I have to say that the months which were particularly difficult for me were April and November. These are the usual months for time change and I often wondered if my brain didn't like that. Coincidentally, April is the month when my mother had her massive psychotic breakdown. November was a tough time for her also. At the beginning of the month, she celebrated her wedding anniversary and my Dad's birthday. They used to go out to eat or to a bar, but then after that she would decline in mood with the approach of the holidays. The holidays always got to her. I have not done an in-depth investigation, but I believe she had more mini-breakdown and hospitalization in April, November and December than any other months. I had a relative who used to climb out of bed and go immediately into a tanning bed for the light before she could function during the day.

Recently, it has been discovered that the change of seasons and Daylight Savings Time has a real impact on people, especially those with Autism, dementia and SAD who have a difficult time adjusting to the circadian disruption. Even in the general population, tempers flare, people are not as alert, learning suffers, cardiovascular events go up, and car accidents are more frequent.

Perinatal Mood and Anxiety Disorders (Postpartum Depression) refers to the anxiety and depression many women suffer during the first year after giving birth. Many people asked if my mother suffered from that disorder. She may have, as I was too young to know how she reacted after my birth and the subsequent births of my four siblings in just 5 years. It is believed that she did not suffer from Postpartum Depression because there was no evidence of it in the five births preceding her Schizoaffective Disorder breakdown, and it usually manifests itself with the first birth. Her diagnosis was a complete psychiatric break involving Schizophrenia and Bi-polar Disorder. If she developed Postpartum Depression with the fifth child, it would have been lost to the psychiatric break that was occurring in the month since the child was born. She did so many suspicious things with the new baby that in this day and age would have raised a red flag for Postpartum Depression, but again all that was secondary to the complete psychotic break which caused her to kill him and his brother.

As I said, there are new disorders coming out all the time and I cannot cover all of them. I hope to have continuing dialogue with the readers to discuss things that may not be covered in the guide or things that need to be further explained.

PSYCHIATRISTS, PSYCHOLOGISTS, THERAPISTS, PMH-APRNS

I am going to say this at the beginning of each of the following categories in this Guide, but I firmly believe that people seeking help for Mental Disease symptoms need to have a brain scan to properly identify where the issues are in their brains BEFORE THEY ARE DIAGNOSED AND GIVEN MEDICATIONS BY A PSYCHIATRIST AND DEFINITELY BEFORE ANY TALK THERAPY BEGINS WITH A PSYCHOLOGIST. Unfortunately, this is not happening for the majority of people nowadays with symptoms of mental illness.

A Psychiatrist is a medical doctor who specializes in mental health, including substance use disorders. They are qualified to assess both the physical and mental aspects of psychological problems. **A Psychiatrist is licensed to prescribe medication.** They diagnose the mental disorders, manage treatment and provide therapy for serious mental issues. An example of the magnitude of the stigma of Mental Disease, is that many Psychiatrists have indicated that they have experienced mental disorders, but most of them said they would be reluctant to disclose this to family, friends or patients. I think there has been some progress discussing Mental Disease more openly and we need that openness to get rid of the stigma. Personally, I would rather be treated by a doctor who has experienced a mental disorder because they have a much better idea of what a person dealing with brain disease is going through.

A Psychologist is not a medical doctor, and **cannot prescribe medication**. Their mission is to provide psychotherapy/ talk therapy to help patients. Talk therapy should not come before a brain scan, a diagnosis and the right medications. It can be a waste of time when the mentally ill person does not have enough clarity to understand what is going on.

I would be lying if I said that things would be better once there was an answer to whether a loved one was going through a temporary personality change or a possible mental issue. As things stand now, without brain scans being done regularly, the diagnoses process is filled with mistakes and hit or miss guesses. The challenge and heartbreak is just beginning in most cases. For those who are looking into finding help for a person with a mental disorder, the journey has just begun and it can be a long and painful one. The medical system is struggling to meet the demands of Mental Disease, and so it will take every bit of effort to remain patient and hopeful, while going through one of the most difficult times in life. I could tell you horror stories, but there is no point to that and the people dealing with Mental Disease are doing their best to get very sick people a more quality life.

I believe that until a mentally diseased person gets a diagnosis from a Psychiatrist who is willing to use brain scans as a tool to determine a cause for the patient's symptoms and can prescribe medication which will help the person feel more positive about life, talk therapy should be put on hold. Again, Dr. Phil in a recent show made it clear that brain scans should be done to look into the brain before talk therapy proceeds.

I do want to make it perfectly clear that the above statement refers specifically to people with Mental Disease who have been diagnosed. Millions of people with all kinds of different issues that have not been diagnosed with a mental disorder, who are trying to cope with life in general, are helped every day by Psychologists and Therapists doing much needed talk therapy. It is the person with serious chemical brain issues, who is in the process of being diagnosed and prescribed medications, who I feel does not benefit from talk/group therapy. It is putting the cart before the horse, and can even cause further complications for the patient's recovery as they are often not in a position to understand what is going on and can misinterpret what is being said.

Getting an appointment with a Psychiatrist can be frustrating, stressful and discouraging, especially when you or someone else is suffering. Make sure to check references and share with people who might be able to recommend someone. If you insist on a brain scan, you may need to do that at a different facility and wait to see a Psychiatrist until the written report is in on the brain scan. This test can save a lot of time and money by going to a Psychiatrist with a definitive diagnoses of what areas of the brain are not functioning properly.

Several members of my group on Facebook, Living with Mental Disease, reminded me about a very important member of the psychiatric community I neglected to include in the Guide. Advanced Practice Psychiatric Nurses (PMH-APRN) who are able to prescribe psychiatric medications in all fifty states. Each state has different requirements for APRNs from full practice authority to needing the permission of a supervising psychiatrist. PMH-CNSs may also prescribe in some states as determined by the individual State Nurse Practices Act. This is important news in view of the fact that Psychiatrists are completely overwhelmed and need all the help they can get.

Advanced Practice Psychiatric Nurses are employed in all areas of the health field and in outpatient and other subspecialties treating mental health disorders. They have a Bachelor's Degree in Nursing and many have Graduate Degrees in psychiatric-mental health nursing. PMH-APRNs are required to re-certify every five years and meet the requirements with clinical practice hours and/or required education classes. I have come to find out they are invaluable members of the psychiatric community.

MEDICATIONS

Every day, people are being prescribed medications for mental disorders based on their own evaluation of how they are feeling. Rather than getting scans of the brain to determine what areas are not functioning correctly, many Psychiatrists rely on blood tests and patient surveys to diagnose Mental Disease. Both blood tests and a person's assessment of what they are going through, is not a safe way to diagnose a disease of an organ in the body. An Oncologist would never suggest a chemotherapy program without doing extensive tests to determine what kind of cancer a person had, where it was, and what stage it was in. The same thing should be true of a disease of the brain.

I made it clear that I firmly believe that mental health medications are the key to a functional life for people with Mental Disease. My life was changed significantly with the first medication I was subscribed. I got lucky that I was diagnosed with only mild depression considering my maternal family history, and that the first medication worked.

It would be totally irresponsible of me to suggest any medications, even though I have extensive experience with the different drugs developed to help with chemical issues in the brain. I know many professionals who are involved in research and clinical trials to give us these drugs and they are my heroes. The process of subscribing a drug is for a Psychiatrist to determine after extensive testing, including a brain scan, and vetting to narrow down what could be the imbalance affecting their patient. Even at that, the process can be complicated until the right drug, or amount of that drug, starts working on the diseased area or areas. In addition, once medication is started, regular blood draws need to be taken to make sure the medication is processing through the body correctly and safely.

What I can discuss with you in laymen's terms is why I believe the right meds are crucial for people with Mental Disease. Medical researchers have found that there are three neurotransmitter areas in the brain which are thought to be defective with Mental Disease, either all together or singularly. Serotonin is one. Norepinephrine is another. Dopamine is another. Defective neurotransmitters do not only cause mental problems, but they are also responsible for many serious health issues.

Serotonin is responsible for sending important signals from one part of the nervous system to another. Some scientists believe it is a hormone as well as a neurotransmitter and that can explain why it can be complicated when it is out of control, especially during puberty and menstruation, and other times when hormones go through changes. The right level of Serotonin is essential for the body to function smoothly, and **if it is too low can result in depression, anxiety, insomnia, and negative thoughts**. Serotonin that is too high can cause severe physical symptoms like muscle rigidity and seizures.

Norepinephrine (noradrenaline) is a neurotransmitter which releases substances to help with skeletal muscle and heart contractions. **It must be working properly to regulate the fight-or-flight syndrome which helps humans cope with acute threats**. Interestingly, researchers believe Norepinephrine also releases hormones in the bloodstream from the adrenal glands. **Problems with the imbalance of norepinephrine levels which are too low are depression, anxiety, PTSD (Post Traumatic Stress Syndrome) and substance abuse. Levels which are too high can cause panic** attacks, hyperactivity, and euphoria, not to mention elevated blood pressure.

Dopamine regulates **the pleasure center of the brain**. If it is not functioning properly, a **person can lose the ability to focus, plan, strive, and generally find any interest or pleasure in all aspects of life.**

My husband has Parkinsons Disease, which attacks the nerves in the neurotransmitters in the brain and unfortunately the nerves in the rest of the body. The health of your nervous system is critical to your well-being. He takes a drug to control the Dopamine level in the brain to helps him maintain some interest and pleasure in life. The drugs that our wonderful research scientists develop help millions of people enjoy a functional existence every single day, and especially those who are mentally ill.

It makes perfect sense to me that a loved one suffering from lack of pleasure in life, inability to plan or focus, mood swings from high to low, panic attacks, anxiety, insomnia, and all of the other symptoms of Mental Disease, **ARE DEFINITELY SUFFERING FROM IMBALANCES IN THE NEUROTRANSMITTERS IN THE BRAIN.**

Right now, testing for levels of chemicals in the neurotransmitters are done with blood and urine samples. Sometimes, the tests are conclusive and a drug can be chosen and started. In other cases, the tests are inconclusive but it does not mean that the person isn't suffering from imbalances in those areas that are not showing up on the tests. This is why I am strongly advocating for brain scans to be the first tool to diagnosing Mental Disease and even the syndrome associated with it. We have too many people spending too much time being diagnosed over and over and medicated over and over because the diagnoses are not right to begin with. We lose so many of them as they struggle to survive year after year with no conclusive diagnosis.

A brain scan would speed up the process of diagnosis and make it easier for the Psychiatrist to determine what disorder his patient is suffering from. It then makes it easier to prescribe the right medication to help the diseased areas in the brain recover.

Even with the brain scan and a quick and conclusive diagnosis, medications which work for one person may not work for another person exhibiting the same symptoms. This is due to the unique metabolism of different individuals. Some people are on two or three different drugs to target the parts of their brain which have been found to be imbalanced.

I would not presume to advise anyone with regard to a drug they should be taking, even though unfortunately I have become familiar with most all of them. What our wonderful medical research scientists do is develop drugs to target imbalances in the brain which are causing people to become mentally ill. Then our dedicated doctors who conduct clinical trials confirm their safety for the general public. They have my deepest respect, as it is an overwhelming job.

Anyone out there who truly believes that a mentally ill person simply has behavioral problems that they need to change in order to get well, need a reality check. The behavioral problems all have explanations in the defects in the brain that control these behaviors. Without the proper medication to stabilize these areas, the behavior will continue.

Today, I had my first experience with someone being admitted for attempted suicide and prescribed an antipsychotic drug. The main symptom of psychosis is that the patient does not understand the difference between what is real and what isn't. They are usually totally out of touch with reality. Sometimes they are experiencing hallucinations and delusions, but not always.

The types of mental disorders which can include psychosis are schizophrenia, schizoaffective disorder, some forms of bipolar disorder, and severe depression. These disorders have already been discussed previously in the guide. I have discovered with research that some psychosis occur outside of any of the above disorders. The anti-psychotic medications, which again I will not mention as it would be totally irresponsible, do calm down both the patient and the neurotransmitters in the brain that are out-of-control so the mental health staff can do their job of helping the patient get well.

Unfortunately, another drug the patient was on was withdrawn cold turkey in a previous hospital stay and resulted in an attempted suicide a few days later. **Again, any withdrawal of a drug cold turkey from a mentally ill person is not medically recommended, unless the drug itself is causing life threatening issues.**

Today, as I add to this section, there is a family paying big bucks to a private institution as a last ditch measure to save their child. The child has attempted suicide three times and been in many hospitals and rehabilitation centers. After only a few days, they are concerned that the care he is receiving is similar to what he got at the other places. The expectation was that they would scan his brain and prescribe medications that would hit the areas that were chemically imbalanced. This child is 19 and if this effort to fix his brain doesn't work, the family is fearful that the child will give up and turn completely to drugs and alcohol to feel better. They were lucky that the child agreed to go to the facility, because even though they have a Power of Attorney it wouldn't have mattered in this place. The person entering the facility has to agree to stay there and not leave.

The child was taken off of a drug within 24 hours of being in the facility, with no explanation to the parents as to why. The last time the patient was removed from a drug, a few days later the police were talking the child down from committing suicide. In conversations with parents, the patient is complaining of not feeling well. Group therapy, activities, social worker meetings, cognitive testing are all available, BUT THEY DO NO GOOD IF THE BRAIN IS BROKEN. This is an example of why I believe that BRAIN SCANS ARE IMPERATIVE FOR DIAGNOSING MENTAL DISEASE, FOLLOWED BY AN ASSESSMENT FROM A PSYCHOLOGIST AS TO WHAT MEDICATIONS WOULD TARGET THE AREAS THAT ARE SHOWING UP WITH CHEMICAL IMBALANCES.

It is pointless to counsel a person suffering from any kind of mental disorder if they are not on the right medications to ease the horrific monsters in their brain. I know that for a fact as I lived with those demons for 50 plus years spending every day doing anything I could to get them out of my life. At 60, I was given a miracle through a clinical trial I didn't even qualify for and put on the right medication to kill the monsters. I wouldn't wish 50 years of dealing with Mental Disease without the right medications on anyone. I can understand why they would turn to alcohol and drugs to fight their demons, as it is often times easier than getting the help they need. The mental health system is overwhelmed and frantically putting a band aid on the problem. It will eventually hit the fan when the band aids all fall off.

After three weeks in the private institution and with brain scans and blood work which finally determined that the patient was so low in serotonin that it was almost undetectable in tests, the patient was put on a medication to increase the serotonin levels in his brain. He is beginning to show some interest in life, a positive sign that his chemical levels are responding to the medications. Hopefully, this will continue. He should have had a brain scan in the other institutions, but unfortunately most do not have the budgets or the inclination to do brain scans.

If the family above was the only one going through the agony of trying to get help for their mentally ill child, that would be one thing, but they are not. Millions and millions of families are suffering every day from the pain of seeing their loved ones try one medication after another with life-threatening side effects like suicidal ideation, and not getting better. Without a definitive brain scan showing where the chemical abnormalities are, prescribing medications will continue to be a hit or miss situation.

I would also be remiss if I didn't mention the fact that most people cannot afford the outrageous costs of brain scans, hospitalization, rehabilitation centers, medications, Psychiatrists, Psychologists, Therapists, and everything else required to treat their disease. We must help people get treatment for Mental Disease, just like we do for Cancer, MS, CF, Diabetes, Kidney Disease, and the thousands of other diseases of the body which are afflicting people. We can't let this remain a silent and stigmatized disease any longer.

HOSPITALIZATION

Hospitalization usually happens when a person attempts suicide, either with our without personal injury. Some go into the Intensive Care Unit if the overdose, gunshot wound, stabbing, or other method chosen to end life requires critical monitoring of physical wounds. Patients who are not injured, are provided a bed and put on constant monitoring for the amount of time dictated by that particular jurisdiction. The length of time usually ranges from 24 hours to 72 hours. Some are recommended to a psych ward or a rehabilitation center, which may or may not be connected to the hospital. Depending on their lot in life and insurance and family issues, they are either fortunate enough to get additional help or walk out and back to their lives, until the next time.

There are other ways mentally ill people enter a hospital other than suicide attempts. Some come in suffering from organ failure due to long term Mental Disease and accompanying addictions. They are picked up off the streets or from homeless shelters, near death. If they manage to survive, they might be out the next day returning to their dysfunctional life. Some enter the hospital because of accidents and injuries due to alcohol and drug addictions used to self-medicate and ease the symptoms from the demons in their brains. If patients have no insurance, chances of going into rehabilitation are slim and none. Beds in rehab are like gold and cost just as much.

If the patient is under 18, the parents will have access to medical information. If the patient is over 18, the parents will be shut out of information unless they have a Power of Attorney. Anyone with a dependent who is showing signs of Mental Disease, needs to get a POA as soon as possible. The mentally ill person needs to agree to the POA and that is where the devastating issues begin, as many won't sign on the dotted line. **It is TRAGIC that parents who are completely supporting a 19 year old who doesn't have the good judgement to take care of themselves, are shut out of critical information on that person.** The system is totally messed up in this regard.

Many people are under the mistaken assumption that hospitals will cure their mentally ill child or adult. That is not the case at all. A mentally ill person needs the help of a licensed PSYCHIATRIST who will evaluate brain scans and blood and urine samples and prescribe the medication or medications they feel has the best possibility of stabilizing the areas of the brain that are not receiving the right amount of chemical stimulus. Depending on the Psychiatrist on duty and his workload at the hospital, which is usually overwhelming, the patient will get initial care and as best a diagnosis as he/she can give during the limited time the patient is in the hospital. Sometimes tests are inconclusive and the patient is referred to other Psychiatrists and clinics for further evaluation.

Your loved one may get lucky while in the hospital and be prescribed just the right medication for their issue, but this outcome is rare and I personally have never heard of a hospital stay which resulted in the patient being cured and not needing additional help when released.

REHABILITATION

By now you know my feelings that the first priority in helping a mentally ill person is to determine where the brain is deficient with SPECT brain scans and blood work. From what I have researched, I believe everyone with Mental Disease needs a SPECT brain scan to determine what areas of the brain are showing signs of dysfunction. Once those results are in and a diagnosis is made, then begins the challenge of finding the right medication for that individual.

Sadly, there is not enough funding resources for the kinds of tests and treatments needed for the number of people who are mentally ill. Brain scans are sometimes not covered under health insurance. Also, rehabilitation begins in most cases before the person is diagnosed or treated with the right medications. On most occasions, the patient has not had the amount of time needed to have a proper diagnosis or be sure the meds are working, and that there are no side effects which would make them feel worse.

At present, most of the diagnoses on people who are mentally ill are made from the surveys given to them. The judgement of a person who is suffering from mental issues is usually very foggy and they are basically being asked to diagnosis themselves. A mentally ill person who is suffering from social distancing, anxiety, inability to communicate, confusion, hostility, and on and on, is not going to do well in a group session with other mentally ill people. They can barely get through one-on-one in most cases. I have witnessed patients becoming very agitated when asked to participate in a survey, questionnaire or interview during a time when they can barely function.

Surveys are a good tool after brain scans and blood work are done and a diagnosis is made, but not a tool to make a diagnosis recommendation. The same goes for all of the activities thought to be important to keep the mentally ill patient "busy". It doesn't work that way as the dysfunctional brain issues are stronger than the ability of the person to override them. The medications must be working to give the patient the ability to feel like participating in life. If they are pushed into action before they are ready, it can result in serious issues like attempted suicide, running away, giving up completely, using drugs and alcohol, and more serious mental issues and psychosis than they had going in due to overload on the brain and feelings of failure and hopelessness.

Many people with several failed rehabilitation stints behind them, and money to afford it, resort to private rehabilitation facilities. Sadly, the majority of people in this world are not able to afford basic rehabilitation. Care must be taken to make sure the facility focuses on diagnosing the correct mental disorder with the best in brain scans and blood tests and then testing the right medications to make sure they are working. Otherwise, you might as well throw your money in the toilet bowel and flush it down.

Until a diagnosis is made and a medication is prescribed to help the brain return to a state where the patient has the ability to be positive about being alive, without struggling every minute of every day to feel that way, no amount of rehabilitation is going to work. I have never heard of a person being healed of a mental disorder by keeping busy and going to group therapy without the benefit of the right diagnosis and medications.

I told you this guide would be about experience, and I have never seen a person with mental disorder symptoms function without medications to regulate their brain. They may "think" they are functioning as they drink their wine and alcohol all day, do their drugs, abuse their loved ones with their anger, mood swings, erratic behavior, compulsive shopping, and on and on, BUT THEY ARE NOT. If I had a dime for every person I have known or talked to who sat through counseling sessions and had no clue what was said, I would be very rich. The abnormalities in the brain need to be attended to first before a person can begin to process therapy. I know three people personally who were undergoing therapy with a Psychologist and a slew of therapists and committed suicide. These specialists could not talk the patient into ignoring their brain's tendency toward suicidal ideation. Only the right diagnosis and medications can do that.

I used to think that rehabilitation was the area in which the mental health system was the most broken, but actually I have discovered it is not (and I will divulge that at the end of this section). Rehabilitation is the area with the most pressure, especially as Mental Disease is increasing and so many people are suffering. Beds are like gold and people needing them sometimes wait in hospital emergency rooms for days and weeks before getting placed. Those people who are not in a hospital, have a very poor chance of getting into a rehab center which does not charge an exorbitant amount of money.

Once a patient has a bed, it may be under the worst conditions for a person suffering from mental issue. I have talked to people who got maybe one or two hours of sleep a night because of all the chaos going on in the wards. Many patients are out-of-control and provide a threatening environment. It is the reason why so many facilities use drugs to sedate the patients, so they can have some order until they can determine what is going on with them. The last thing a mentally ill person needs is no sleep, but the facilities are often not conducive to a peaceful environment.

The law is that 18 year olds are adults, even if they are being completely supported by their family. A family goes through unimaginable pain being separated from their child and being cut out of all decision-making, test results, and treatment. Parents have had to get emergency Power of Attorney paperwork to gain control over a child. Some get their child to cooperate, while others have to collect documentation from doctors and hire expensive lawyers to declare their child unable to make decisions for themselves. The cost is formidable, on top of whatever they are putting out for Psychiatrists, medications, and the rehabilitation center. Most insurances are very limited as to what they will pay for what they consider to be "behavioral issues". This is pathetic when you consider that the brain is diseased and causing mental issues. It is the same as the disease of cancer which causes many parts of the body, including the brain, to malfunction. Many people get brain scans to diagnose cancer and they are covered by insurance. The coverage should be the same for brain scans to diagnose Mental Disease.

There is no way a child who is being fully supported by parents or family can be considered an adult, especially if they are also suffering from Mental Disease. Something needs to be done to give parents the ability to get control quickly, but presently they must hire a lawyer to go to court to protect the best interests of their child.

I am sorry to say that I don't have much hope in the current climate that this will ever be rectified. Prepare to be frustrated and overwhelmed, but this is another area where you need to ask for help from people who have had experience with different facilities. Again, in most cases the mentally ill person goes wherever there is a bed available. By this time in the process of following the Plan of Action and getting to the point of rehabilitation, family members are relieved to have whatever time they can to recover from the trauma of what has happened. Any facility seems fine as long as they know their child is under lockdown and surveillance. I know it is hard to believe the situation could deteriorate to that point, but it often does. It is nothing to be ashamed of and is actually a necessary break for caretakers to focus on self-care and recuperation for what might be to come.

A young man of 19 who was lucky enough to go into a private facility was given extensive blood tests and a brain scan after a week at the facility. It was discovered his serotonin level was almost non-existent and that his dopamine level was too high. He was put on new medications that hopefully will help normalize those levels. These levels might have been the case from the very beginning of his ordeal or it might be the result of incorrect levels of medication over the long period of time he has been mentally ill. They also noted that his metabolism level for the drugs he is being given is very rapid. The way a person metabolizes drugs is critical as it determines the amount of the drug which needs to be given daily to work most effectively to stabilize the patient.

Further tests will be done because the young man has experienced head and eye injuries in his life from sports, which could have caused Traumatic Brain Injury (concussions, orbital injuries, etc.). The area of the brain that is most likely impacted by TBI is the frontal cortex, where blood does not flow correctly, causing malfunctions in the chemical neurotransmitters. In other words, important chemical nerve transmitters in the brain (dopamine, serotonin, etc.) are not getting the right stimulation to function properly. Actually, I am told TBI cannot really be diagnosed with any tests out nowadays and that the only conclusive diagnosis is with an autopsy. There are areas of the brain that may light up in tests like the SPECT but they will not determine if the defective area is because of Mental Disease or TBI. Again, it really doesn't matter because TBI is treated the same as other mental disorders, depending on what area of the brain is malfunctioning. Unfortunately, at this point the SPECT brain scan is not offered in most hospitals or rehabilitation centers.

In the meantime, I am told every day seems to bring more clarity to the young person, but the person is still not able to say they are feeling positive about life on a day-to-day basis without struggling. It is critical that enjoying life on a day-to-day basis comes naturally without struggling, before success can be celebrated.

Recently, the above patient was moved to another rehabilitation facility which focuses on preparing people diagnosed with Mental Disease and addiction issues the life skills they need to get back out in the world. Presumably, the other facility found the right medication to stabilize the lack of serotonin which was missing in his brain and the patient is ready for the next step in the plan. The cost of this entire process would be prohibitive for the majority of people with Mental Disease.

It is sad that this person is one of the few who is fortunate enough to have the benefit of very expensive treatment to help fix his brain. Unfortunately, the majority of people suffering from Mental Disease will never see the inside of a hospital, rehab center, psychiatric office, psychologist, therapist or medication in their lifetime.

The end goal for everyone dealing with the mentally ill, including the mentally ill person themselves, is to get to the point where the loved one, child, parent, friend or neighbor can say, *I feel positive about life and optimistic about living on a daily basis without struggling to feel that way.* Only then can we be sure the medications are working and that the person can live a functional life. It was the best day of my life when the cloud of Mental Disease lifted from me. I was able to function with my mild depression during life until the age of 60, but it wasn't easy and definitely not quality of life. It is no way for a person to live. I wish I had a Plan of Action to follow back then.

You will remember I told you that I believe rehabilitation is not the most broken part of the mental health system at this time, so I owe you an answer as to what I think is fractured. I believe the method of diagnosing Mental Disease is no longer acceptable, and that brain scans are needed for all people suffering with Mental Disease symptoms as a FIRST LINE OF DIAGNOSIS. It is archaic to diagnose a person without looking at their brain first and determining what areas are not working. It is irresponsible to diagnose them based on their own evaluations of themselves and blood tests which are not conclusive. Many mental health syndromes do not even have markers in the blood to detect them. Blood tests are important tools AFTER the person is on the right medications to determine if they are metabolizing them correctly, but should not be a way to make a diagnosis. They are just too inconclusive and unreliable for such a critical and important part of the diagnostic process.

If a person was seeing a doctor for possible cancer, the Oncologist would not diagnose them based on how they were feeling or from one blood test. There are a myriad of physical exams and specialized blood tests which are done before there is any attempt to treat the person. Every organ which could possibly be involved is x-rayed and studied. Why should this be any different for a Mental Disease of the brain? The brain must be scanned and studied first.

CONCLUSION

1. If you, a family member or friend are undergoing a personality change, follow the PLAN OF ACTION immediately.

2. I believe a BRAIN SCAN is the first necessary step to diagnose areas of the brain which are showing signs of damage. This can avoid months and years of a misdiagnosis and the wrong medications being prescribed. I realize this is out of reach for most people, but hoping the access to this diagnostic scan will change in the future. If a brain scan is not possible, please make an appointment with a Psychiatrist, PMH-APRN, Psychologist, or Therapist as soon as possible. Some people can do very well functioning with mental health issues with talk therapy.

3. Only a PSYCHIATRISTS or PMH-APRN is licensed to diagnose mental illness and to prescribe drugs which have been developed to help regulate chemicals in the brain that are causing mental illness.

4. Being prescribed the RIGHT MEDICATION for a chemical imbalance in the brain is critical. Never stop a prescribed medication without a Psychiatrists approval.

5. It is putting the cart before the horse expecting a mentally ill person to benefit from talk therapy before the brain is regulated with medicines and they can process what they are being told. Unfortunately, in this day and age the

medical profession has a tendency to prescribe them both at the same time. Again, some people have mental health issues which respond very well to talk therapy alone.

6. Never leave children alone with a person who is exhibiting abnormal behavior. Actually, there are not many people of any age who would do well against a person who is out-of-control.

7. Never antagonize a person who is exhibiting abnormal behavior. Get help immediately.

8. If a person living in your home is behaving abnormally and refuses to cooperate with attempts to help them, you must be prepared to enforce tough love and do whatever it takes to remove them from your environment before they do harm.

9. Don't keep mental health issues to yourself for fear of stigma and shame. Mental illness is a disease just like cancer, and needs serious treatment. Try to find out from family if there are hereditary issues involving Mental Disease.

10. Be prepared for frustration with all aspects of trying to get help for Mental Disease, but do not give up.

11. Educate people as often as you can about Mental Illness being a legitimate disease of the brain.

12. Visit my Facebook group, Living with Mental Disease, to discuss further issues with mental illness. For example, coping mechanisms such as walking, meditation,

journaling, lowering expectations, distracting the brain, talking to people, and ways of keeping the brain healthy are discussed in depth in the posts.

I am realizing as administrator of my recently established group on Facebook, Living with Mental Disease, that this illness is rampant in our society. There are never-ending questions which people are asking not only on the site but with calls, e-mails and messages. We must do everything we can to educate people about the disease and help reduce the stigma so people are more comfortable asking for help.